# AMAZING GRACE

VENETIA SHERSON

# AMAZING GRACE

♡ ♡ ♡

A story of surrogacy and the
love of two New Zealand sisters

First published 2021

JAG Publishing

ISBN 978-0-473-57876-3

Designed by Enni Tuomisalo
Typeset in PT Serif, 10 pt

**Disclaimer**
While this book is intended as a general information resource and all care has been taken in compiling the contents, neither the author nor the publisher and their distributors can be held responsible for any loss, claim or action that may arise from reliance on the information contained in this book. As each person and situation is unique, it is the responsibility of the reader to consult a qualified professional regarding their personal care.

*To Maddy, who made our family complete, and Karene who helped bring Grace Madeleine Sherson into the world in the most perfect way.*

# Contents

PROLOGUE

# The Worst Day

*Breathe, she tells herself. Just breathe. But breath won't come. She tries to focus. The specialist is explaining the next steps. She hears the words "urgent" and "essential." The specialist shows a picture of a cone biopsy of her cervix and pinpoints where the abnormal cells have spread. She hears her mother, a barrister, asking probing questions in the way she would of witnesses in court. "What are her options? There must be an alternative. What can we do?" She sees her sister, watching her. Keeping her safe with her eyes. Telling her silently, this will be all right. We will get through this together. She trusts her sister more than anyone else in the world. They have been besties since childhood. She wants to believe her. But two words are on rotate in her brain.*

*No babies.*

*She is 31 years old, a lawyer, newly in love, planning a life together, a family.*

*No babies.*

On the drive home, her sister holds her in her arms while her mother manoeuvres the car through motorway traffic. She thinks now how hard that must have been and of her mother's reassuring focus on solutions. She remembers cars passing through a blur of tears. Feeling overwhelmed and disconnected. And angry. "Why me?" she asks over and over. And then, the universal mantra of those faced with devastating news: "It's just not fair."

It takes two hours to travel from Greenlane Hospital in Auckland to Hamilton. They drive straight to her mother's house and she dials her partner's phone. "Can you come?" When he arrives minutes later, her mother and sister leave them alone. It's a warm spring day and they sit by the pool. There are the sounds of children playing in the park opposite. "Babe, it's the worst news," she says. "The cancer is aggressive. They need to do a radical hysterectomy within a month in case it spreads further. That means I can't have children." Then she buries her head in his chest and weeps. He holds her and strokes her hair. He talks about her health being more important to him than fertility. "It'll be okay, babe," he says. She doesn't believe it then. But she feels his strength will get them through...

# CHAPTER 1

# An epiphany in
# the jungle

In 2015, Jemani Alchin-Boller sat with her friend Dani in the lotus position on the roof of their tiny wooden cabin in the Costa Rican rainforest, looking at the moon and trying to figure out her life. The air was thick with the croaks of red-eyed tree frogs and the chirps and rustles of other creatures going about their nightly business. It was a new moon, too pale to see far into the jungle, but the women had hauled an old lamp up a ladder through the loft, along with a bottle of Argentinian Malbec. The lamp illuminated their faces, their hair loosely knotted, hands in a mudra position – index fingers lightly touching their thumbs. The moon's fine crescent made the stars look brighter and the sky darker. Jem closed her eyes. She was 30; she had a law degree; she had travelled for two years, non-stop, supervising busloads of hormone-fuelled backpackers around Europe. She had walked out of a relationship after eight years, finally understanding it was unhealthy for both of them. She had imagined her life taking shape like a jigsaw puzzle, the pieces neatly interlocked. But everything felt fragmented and uncertain. Back home in New Zealand, friends were mostly married, planning babies and new curtains. She met them for coffee and drinks but felt out of place in their world. "Have you met anyone?" they asked, stunned that their beautiful friend was still single. "When are you going to begin practising law?" It was the same questions she asked herself, along with, "What *do* I want from my life?"

It was Dani's idea to come up on the roof. Dani was a life coach and on her own journey of self-discovery. She was two years younger than Jem, single without kids and moving from country to country working from her computer on charity projects. She viewed the moon as an ally in finding answers to the Big Questions and saw it could be helpful to her friend. "A new moon is rejuvenating," she said as they clambered up the ladder, balancing the Malbec and the lamp. "A time for new beginnings."

The new moon contemplation included a ritual that involved writing down a list of things to let go of, then burning it. When the negative thoughts had been seen off, new intentions could be set in play. The approach made sense to Jem and, in a rich jungle setting with an edge-of-the world feeling, it felt like a good place to jump off.

When Dani had suggested Jem join her in Costa Rica, Jem was weighing up whether to attend a wedding in Hawaii. She worked out she could have six weeks in Costa Rica for the same price as a wedding outfit and a hotel for a few days in Honolulu. Time with her friend seemed an ideal escape from a life that was rapidly settling into a humdrum round of work, study and admiring other couple's babies. She stored her stilettos and suits at her mother's house, booked a flight from Auckland to San Jose, then jumped on a tiny plane that landed on a grass runway in the middle of the jungle, the closest landing strip to Santa Teresa, a tiny hamlet near the southern tip of the Nicoya Peninsular, peppered with yoga retreats and organic eateries. The town is nirvana for surfers, big-city drop-outs, and the odd celebrity on a detox diet. The most common expression is "pura vida" which translates as "simple life". The biggest concern for locals – "Ticos" – is whether to pave the bumpy, dusty track that serves as the main road. It was May when Jem arrived and the temperature was in the mid-30s. Swathes of mist hung about the forest and she could hear monkeys jabbering in the trees. Quad bikes were lined up to take the new arrivals into town. Jem heaved her too-full backpack from the plane and jumped on a bike behind a bare-backed local.

The house where Dani lived was a small square two-storeyed building divided into two flats. Dani lived in the upstairs flat. Two Americans who owned a tattoo parlour lived below, surfing, and smoking dope when they weren't engraving "pura vida" on departing travellers' arms. Jem and Dani shared a bed, except when Dani's boyfriend stayed over, when she moved to the couch. Her days settled into an easy pattern, beginning at dawn when she walked a few metres to the beach, sucked in the sea air, wrote in her diary, and listened to Jack Johnson and Ed Sheeran on her phone. She jotted down random thoughts and tried not to beat herself up for not having answers to all life's questions. She practised yoga with a gentle grey-haired yogi who talked about life as a process in a constant state of change.

The contrast with her previous life could not have been greater. As a tour-guide, her life had been fast-paced and party-fuelled: sky-diving in Austria, bungy-jumping in Croatia, toga parties in Rome and a lot of alcohol. Between co-ordinating arrivals and departures in European cities and dishing out advice and cures for hangovers and broken hearts, she would collapse in her London flat desperate for solitude and sleep. In Costa Rica she found time for contemplation and reflection. Did she want to continue to travel? Where would she settle? Henry Miller wrote, "One's destination is never a place, but a new way of seeing things." It was a philosophy tailor-made for a young woman a long way from home, in the throes of a quarter-life crisis. As the weeks passed, she could feel her mind calming. Her senses became heightened; colours seemed more vivid; sounds and smells more pronounced. She went on a cleansing diet, showered in the rain, and slept like a baby. No one asked what she did. They were interested only in her ideas. When she saw a sign for a legal firm in town, she briefly toyed with the idea of staying there for ever.

Six weeks after she arrived, she and Dani jumped on a quad bike and travelled for hours along a dusty coastal road. They dismounted and sat cross-legged on a cliff high above the bright Pacific Ocean. The jungle stretching into the distance was so dense it looked black. Jem focused on the surf below and thought, could this be enough? A place where no plan extended beyond tomorrow; where there were no pressures to practise law, buy a house or start a family? Could she retreat forever? But nearly 12,000km away, where the Pacific also lapped New

Zealand's shores, was family. She missed her mother's lawyer-honed debates around the dinner table; her father's calm counsel, and her youngest brother's desperate pleas for help when an assignment was due. Most of all, she missed her sister, the person she loved most in the world. As the sun began to sink, changing the sky from apricot to crimson, she turned to her friend. "It's time for me to leave."

        ♥     ♥     ♥

Maddy Turner was getting her daughter Amelia ready for school when she learned her sister was coming home. While Jem was in Costa Rica they had kept in touch through Skype, but Maddy missed her. She knew Jem was unsettled when she left New Zealand. She referred to her departure as a "fuck-it" moment. "Jem had been living this high life in Europe for two years, and when she came home to finish her professionals to be admitted to the bar, she was well over being a poor student again. She wasn't in a relationship. We were all nesting. She wanted to go out but a lot of our friends had left town and she had no wing women. She was in a bit of a funk before she left to stay with Dani."

Maddy's life had taken a different route to Jem's. She met her future husband, Joe, when they were both high school students – she at Hillcrest High, which Jem had also attended, and he at Melville High on the other side of the city. They might never have met but for a traumatic incident in 2003, when Maddy was 15. A car driven by a drugged 18-year-old – the designated driver of a group of friends – smashed into a telegraph pole, killing a 17-year-old passenger, and gravely injuring his girlfriend – Maddy's best friend – and several others. Over the summer following the accident, Maddy effectively moved in to her friend's house during her recovery. Joe was the best friend of the injured young woman's brother and part of the group that gathered at the house. Their friendship deepened and, at the end of 2004, Joe took her to meet his beloved grandparents who he lived with. Maddy saw the way he cared for his grandad. She liked that they shared the same values and commitment to family. She did not know then how those values would impact on the decisions they would later have to make.

In 2007, she and Joe travelled to Australia. Joe had completed his apprenticeship in welding in stainless steel fabrication and the couple was keen to travel. They went to the Gold Coast for 18 months and then to Murrindindi in Victoria, before heading to the Sunshine Coast. In 2010, when Maddy was 24, they travelled to Perth where Maddy found she was pregnant. She was shocked at the timing, but secretly delighted. She was from a family of four and had always known she wanted children. In June, their daughter, Amelia, was born by Caesarean section at Perth Hospital, weighing 3.8kg. The labour wasn't long, but the birth was traumatic. Maddy felt bullied by staff who she says pressured her into an unnecessary intervention. She was heavily sedated and struggled to breastfeed her daughter. When she took her home from hospital, five days later, she felt exhausted and overwhelmed. "I had Mum and Joe's parents there, and Jem, who was living with us at the time, but when they left, it felt different. Our friends in Perth were still living the party lifestyle. We weren't. We'd been away for five years, plus both our families were in New Zealand." They decided to return.

In New Zealand, following her experience of a hospital birth in Perth, Maddy began studying to be a midwife and, in 2012, she and Joe married. When she became pregnant with her second child, she resolved the birth would be different, and set about preparing for a homebirth.

Pursuing a natural (vaginal) birth after a C-section (VBAC) is not without risk. Some doctors are reluctant to proceed because there is a chance the uterus could rupture. During Amelia's birth, Maddy had also been labelled CPD (cephalo-pelvic disproportion), which means a baby's head or body is too large to fit through the mother's pelvis. Second babies can be bigger than firstborns, so she could have been persuaded that an elected Caesarean was her best option. But the memories of her hospital birth in Perth were raw, and the benefits of a natural homebirth compelling. In her midwifery training, she had attended around a dozen births and seen a range of experiences. She had also done her research and knew a vaginal birth presented fewer potential complications than surgery. She was not concerned by the prospect of a long labour and relished the thought of giving birth at her home, supported by family. She engaged experienced Hamilton midwife Karene Clark, who had done several VBACs and was supportive of her choice. And then she waited.

On May 24, 2014, six days after his expected date, Lachlan Laurance (after Joe's grandfather) Turner, was born at home, weighing 4.2kg (500gm more than his sister, and with a head circumference 2cm larger, dispelling the idea that Maddy's babies could not fit through the birth canal). The labour lasted three days. Jem, who had returned to New Zealand from Europe to complete her professionals, took turns with Joe and Rose, rubbing her sister's back, offering encouragement. Jem cried as she held her new-born nephew in her arms. Watching them, Maddy also wept. She knew then her sister was destined to be a mum. When Jem came back from Costa Rica the following year, that view was affirmed. "Jem was glowing with good health. But there was something else. She had had this experience with Dani, who was a bit of an Earth Mother, and she was inspired to make changes. She had sorted out a lot of stuff that she needed to let go of. It was a sort of an 'Eat, Pray, Love' moment." Jem talked openly about her dream to have a baby of her own. Maddy secretly hoped she would meet a man with similar ideas.

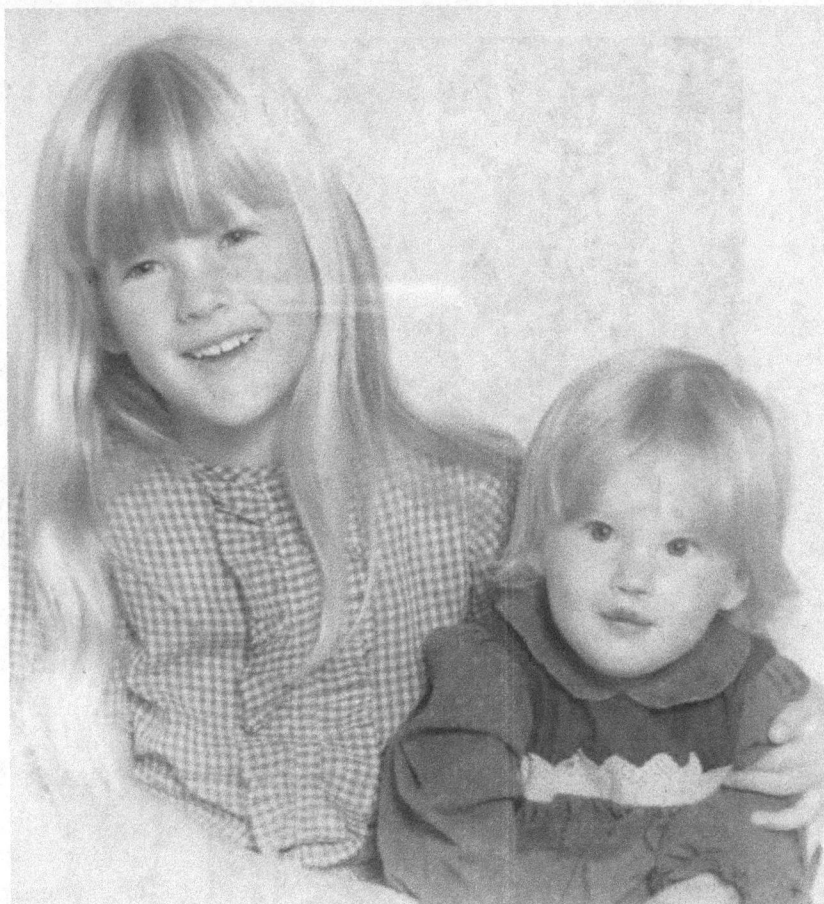
Big sister, little sister: Jem, left, aged 4 and Maddy, 1.

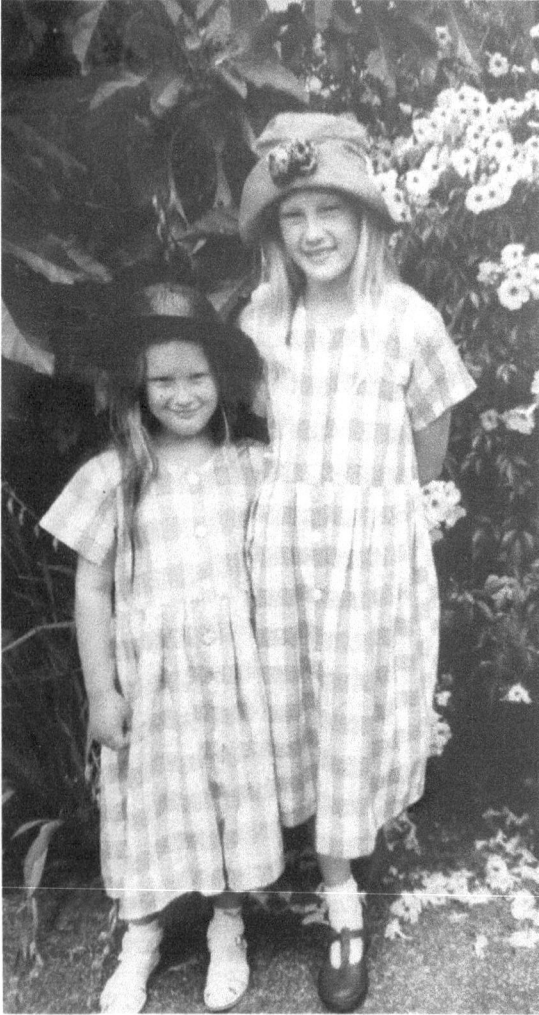

Growing up. Rose says her daughters have different personalities, "but they are always in each other's corner."

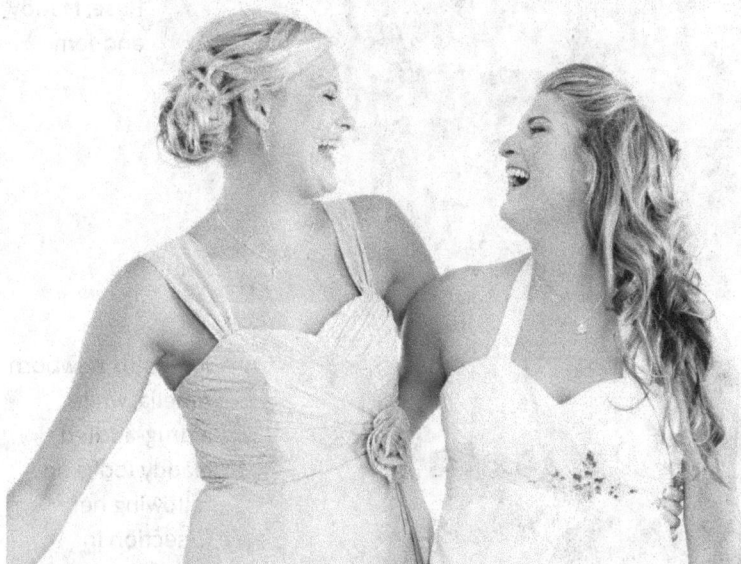

Wedding belles. Jem was Maddy's best woman at her marriage to Joe in December 2012.

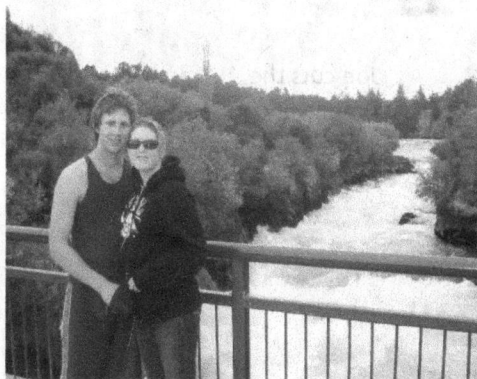

Young love. Maddy met Joe when they were at school after Maddy and her best friend were involved in a fatal accident.

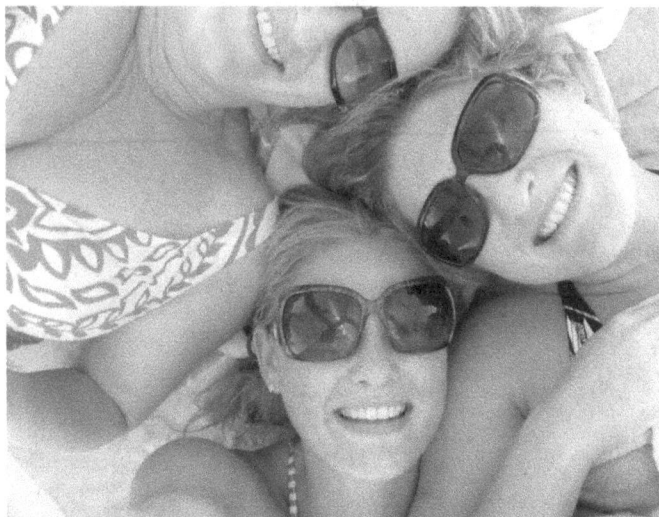

The Alchin women have always been close. From left, clockwise: Rose, Maddy and Jem

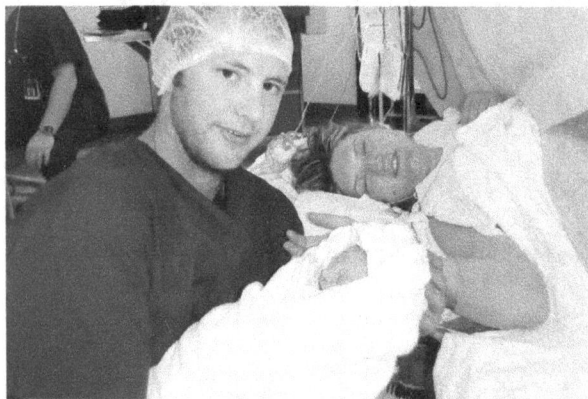

Joe holds newborn Amelia, while a drug-addled Maddy looks on following her C-section in Australia.

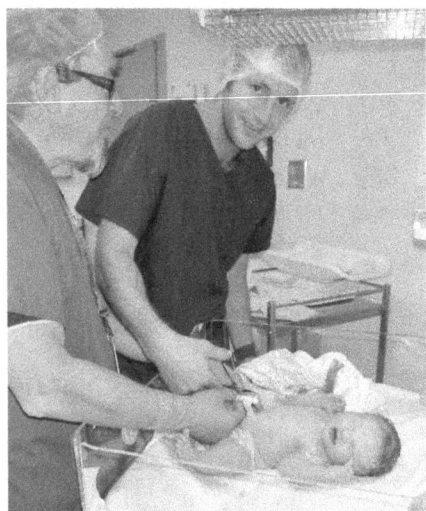

Joe cuts the umbilical cord, watched by the obstetrician.

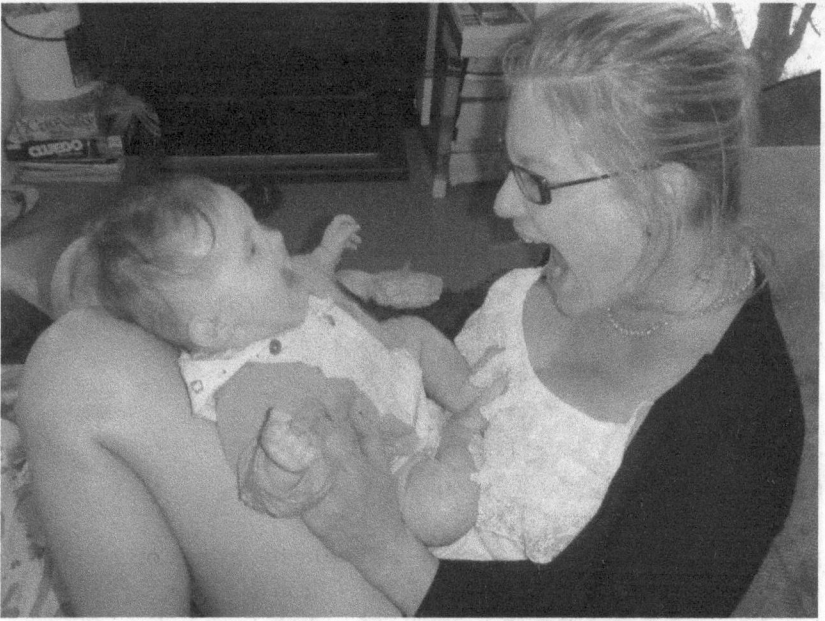

Aunty Jem with baby Amelia. Jem has always had a close relationship with her niece and nephews.

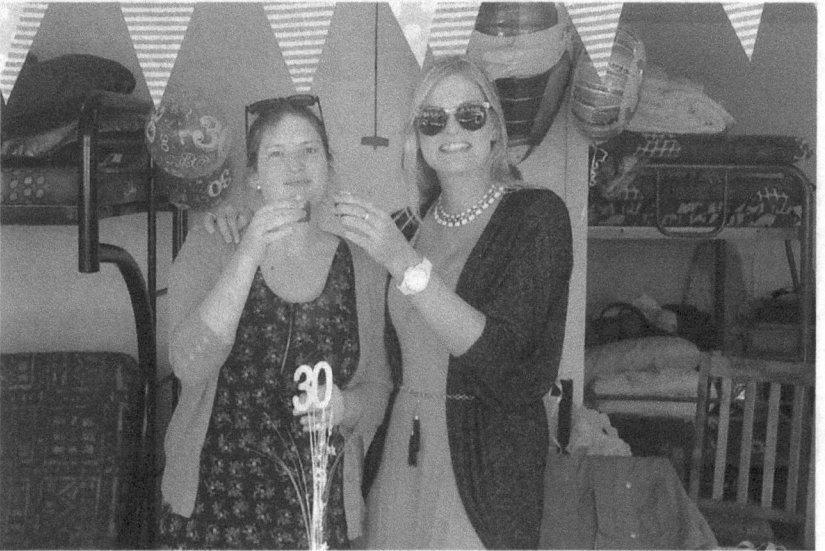

The 'fuck-it' moment. Jem and Maddy party before Jem heads to Costa Rica to look for answers.

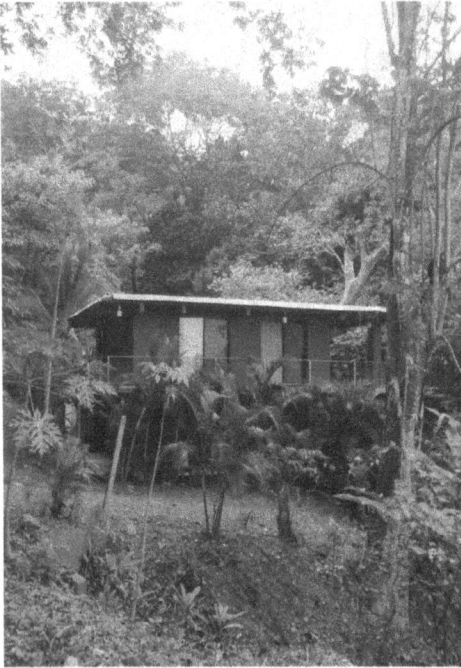

The hut in the Costa Rican rainforest, where Jem and her friend Dani lived.

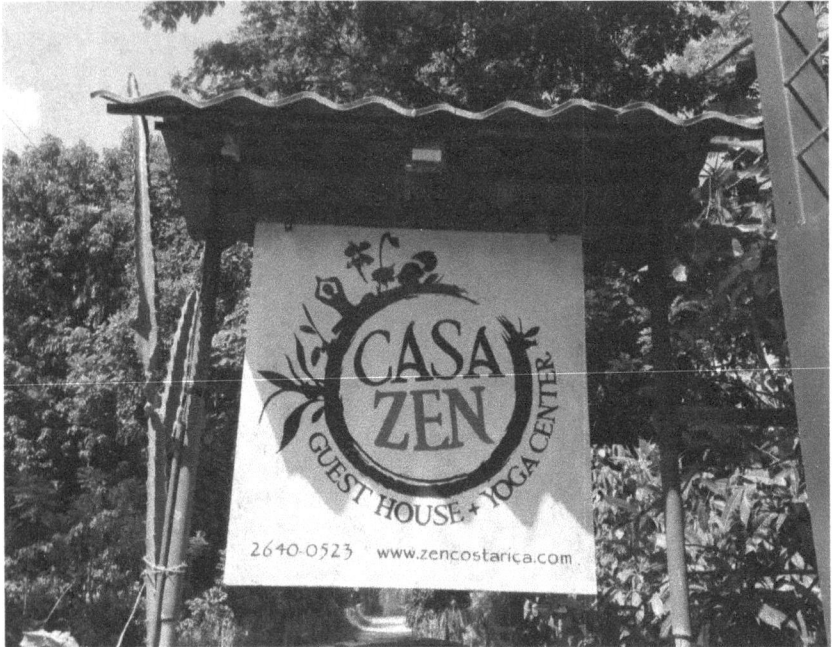

The yoga centre where Jem practised meditation and thought about the big questions in her life.

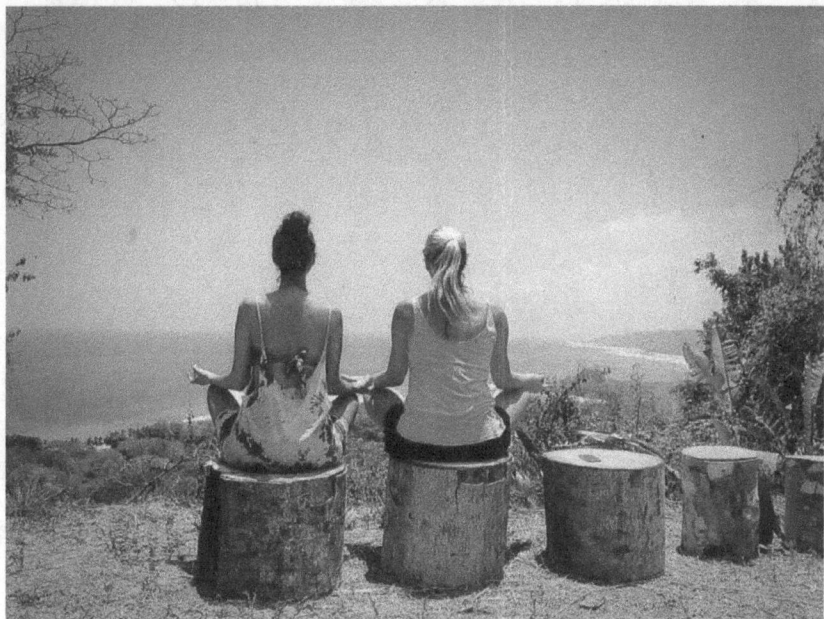

Jem and Dani meditate high above the Pacific Ocean. It was the moment when Jem knew she had to leave.

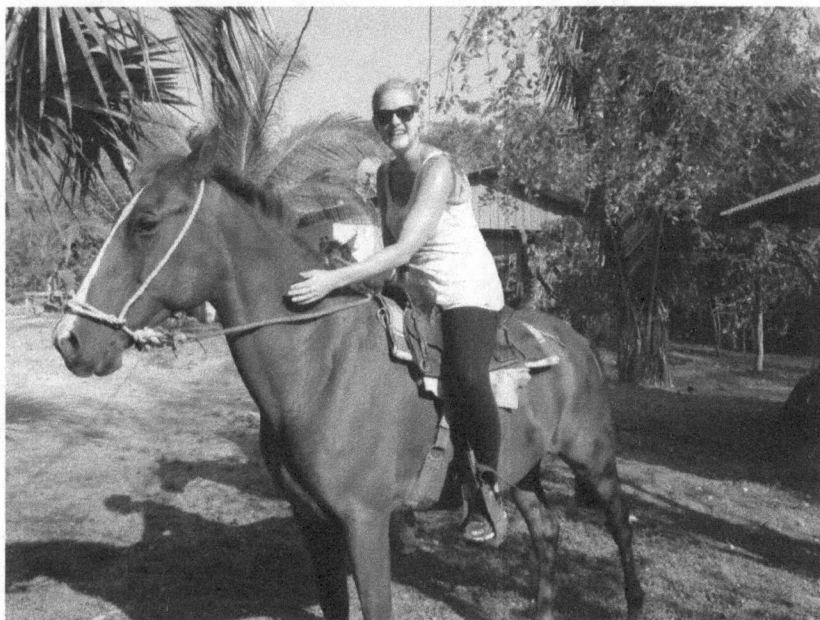

Jem heads off for a ride along the beach at Santa Teresa in Costa Rica.

# CHAPTER 2

# Jem meets her soulmate

On June 19, 2015, the day of her admission to the bar, Jem was in excellent spirits, relieved to have finally completed her qualifications, which she had begun five years before. To her mother's amusement, she insisted on wearing her wig and gown all day. Rose had been delighted when Jem elected to study law, after initially considering business studies. She felt her elder daughter was well-suited to the profession. "She has an analytical mind and she's without doubt the most articulate person I know," she says. "When she knows what she wants she really goes for it." The hour-long ceremony was conducted at the High Court at Hamilton. Rose was her daughter's moving counsel and the court was filled with family, friends, and Rose's colleagues. Afterwards, the group decamped to Gothenburg, a popular tapas restaurant in Hamilton beside the Waikato River. At some stage, Jem's former schoolmate Robbie Oxenham joined the gathering. He had rung earlier to ask if he could bring a mate, another friend from Hillcrest High. Jem knew Mark Sherson from school, but he was slightly older, not part of her close network of friends. The couple chatted briefly over lunch, Jem still wearing her buttoned-up white shirt, wig, and gown; her blonde hair neatly tied back from her face. Later, the group went back to Rose's house to continue the celebration. As the evening wore on, she and Mark continued to talk. Jem was openly flirty. "He really caught my eye."

A week later, the pair met again at a Hamilton pub, with a group of friends. Mark had also come out of a long relationship, but at the time he was single and living in Hillcrest with his 16-year-old son, Ethan, who was in his last year at school. He invited Jem to a meal at their house, and she liked the way the father and son got on. She knew from the outset this would be more than just a casual fling. A chance encounter with a fortune teller at a friend's birthday party seemed to confirm that. "She [the fortune-teller]

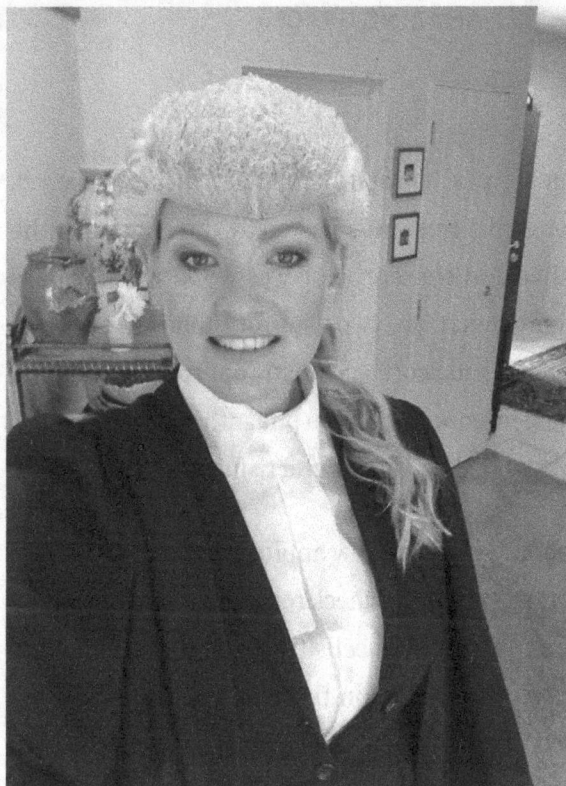

Admission to the bar. Rose says her daughter is well-suited to the profession because of her analytical mind.

told me my grandfather, who had died some years before, had communicated my boyfriend was 'the one.' She also told me I had to let my guard down. 'He (Mark) is 100 per cent there, but you are not', she said. Mark's response, when she relayed that news was, "Oh, God." But secretly he was pleased. He was devoting his energy to his landscaping business and raising Ethan, but he knew the woman in his life was special. Maddy was also at the birthday party. The fortune teller told her she was trying to have another baby, which was far from her mind.

Over the next four months, Jem and Mark's relationship deepened. They went on long bike treks and walked by the sea and in the bush. Jem felt alive and content. She was working three days a week as a data processor and two days for Hamilton barrister Scott McKenna. She liked Scott's altruistic approach to helping the little guy, which fitted with her own philanthropic philosophy. All the fears that she had had about practising law disappeared.

In October in keeping with her new approach to healthy living, she had a smear test – a routine check recommended for women every three years that removes cells from the cervix to detect any abnormalities. After being on the road in Europe for two years, Jem wanted to get back into a regular routine. She wasn't worried; she had no symptoms and felt well. She reassured Mark it was just a precautionary procedure and they put it out of their minds. The following day the doctor's surgery asked her to return immediately for further tests. "I thought they had made a mistake," she said. But she also felt first twinge of anxiety. After the second test she received a phone call that would change her life.

❤  ❤  ❤

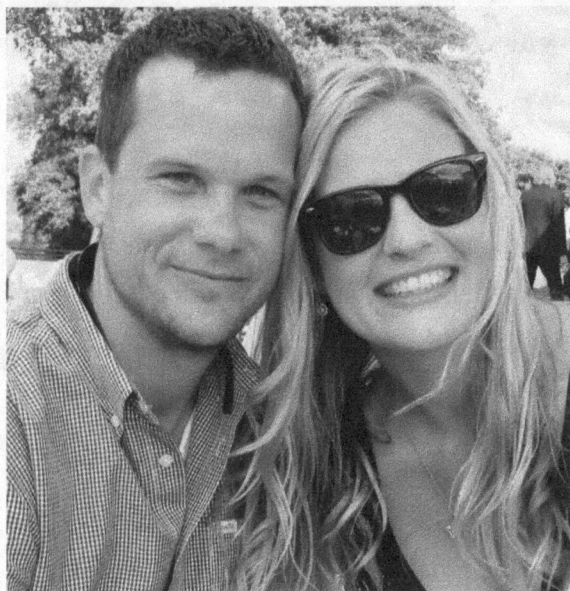

Jem meets Mark, the man she will later describe as her "true north."

Cervical cancer is an insidious disease. It can take years to develop and often there are no symptoms. It is caused by the human papillomavirus HPV, which is sexually transmitted. Most women diagnosed with pre-cancerous changes are in their twenties and thirties, but the average age of women diagnosed with cervical cancer is the mid-fifties. In New Zealand around 160 women are diagnosed each year.

Jem's cancer was at Level 3. At that level, the cancerous cells may have spread throughout the pelvic area. She was given an urgent appointment with a gynaecologist at Waikato Hospital. When she phoned Maddy from her car, she couldn't speak for tears. Maddy said, "I'll come with you. We're doing this together." The next day, she held Jem's hand while the doctor inserted into her cervix a wire loop through which an electrical current is passed to remove abnormal cells. The specialist warned her it wouldn't be pleasant. Jem looked up at the ceiling where there was a painting of a bright blue sky. "Try to float away," said Maddy, squeezing her hand. "Don't think about what is going on." But she could smell the burning flesh.

The following day, she drove to Taupō with her boss, Scott. The trip took her mind off what was happening. She was looking forward to a quiet weekend with Mark. On the return trip, along a new stretch of highway between Cambridge and Hamilton, her phone buzzed again. The hospital wanted her to return for another urgent appointment after the weekend. "It suddenly hit me. I couldn't think where I was or where I was driving to. I thought, 'I shouldn't be driving'." When she arrived at the law office, her workmates were appalled she would have to live with the uncertainty over the weekend and urged her to seek an appointment that day. A new doctor confirmed her fears. She needed to have a cone biopsy to see how far the cancer had spread. Rose, who was with her, started crying. "Mum doesn't cry often," Jem said. "I knew this must be bad." Rose had initially not been worried by the tests. She knew many women had false readings and that, if abnormal cells were detected, they could be treated by laser surgery, a procedure that took only a few minutes. "I thought, 'it's a treatable disease'." As the news got worse, she became increasingly worried, but still held to the hope that the cancer had been detected early enough to offer a range of options. Hospital staff were also reassuring. A few days before Christmas, the cone biopsy was completed and Jem and Mark headed to her father's home at Whitianga on the Coromandel Peninsula to wait for the results.

The Coromandel Peninsula is one of New Zealand's most tranquil beauty spots with dark forests and sugar-sanded beaches. Over the summer months, the population swells as thousands kick back at their beach houses, enjoying the simple pleasures of beachball and barbecues. Normally, Mark would have gone fishing with Jem's dad, Henry, a retired psychologist. They would have had fresh snapper, washed down with a cold beer, and played games with Maddy and Joe's two kids, who adored their Aunty Jem. But the young couple was stressed and distracted. They went for long walks alone on the beach and through the bush, trying to calm their nerves, while they waited for the phone call. Jem tried to focus on the beauty of her surroundings to stop her mind from spiralling. She tried to envisage a phone call with good news. When it came, she stood on the deck of her father's home staring out to sea. The cancer had been detected near the margins of the cervix, where the uterus begins. An urgent appointment was scheduled at Auckland's Greenlane Hospital.

From inside the house, Maddy watched her sister take in the news. She knew Jem was desperately anxious that treatment could affect her fertility. She also knew she had to impart her own news at the worst possible time. The fortune teller had been right. She was seven weeks' pregnant, a pregnancy unplanned, but still joyous. When the kids had been put to bed, she sat down beside her sister. "I've got something to tell you," she said. And then she burst into tears. For Jem it was bittersweet news. "It felt horrible that Maddy felt bad in having to tell me. I was overjoyed for her. She should have been overjoyed in telling me. But I could see how bad she felt." She held her sister in a bear hug and cried with her. With so much going on, the impact of the news did not hit home. She had not yet let her mind go to a place where having her own child might not be an option. The full realisation of her sister's impending birth and her own childlessness only came months later when she reached her lowest ebb.

# CHAPTER 3

# 'there's no easy way to say this...'

On a warmer-than-average summer day in January 2016, Dr Michelle Harris sat in her office at Greenlane Hospital in Auckland and waited for her patient to arrive. Australian by birth, she had been at Greenlane for just a few months, recruited from London where she had completed a six-year fellowship in gynaecological oncology and robotic surgery. A talented pianist, with a degree in music, she had chosen instead to pursue medicine, and to specialise in obstetrics and gynaecology. She was particularly interested in young women with cancer so it was no surprise, when she met with three other specialists at a group clinic in Auckland, that she picked up Jem's file.

While she had not met the young woman who was about to come through her door, she knew her medical background intimately from the data compiled by the multi-disciplinary medical team over several months. "It's a bit topsy-turvy," she says. "You don't get to meet the person involved at the outset. In effect, we know their story and make a recommendation for treatment before we get to meet them. It's odd, because clearly the person to make the decision about treatment is the patient." She would like to change that.

The case notes said the patient had a 1B1 adenocarcinoma cervical cancer, which is less common than squamous cell cancers in the cervix, but generally treated in the same way. The cone biopsy carried out in Hamilton had shown the tumour was just over 2cm, and close to the edge of the uterus. There were several treatment options for the clinical team to weigh up. For 1B1 tumours, the standard surgical treatment is a radical hysterectomy, which includes removal of the uterus and cervix, radical resection of the parametrial tissue and upper vagina, and removal of lymph nodes in the pelvic area. Another option, used to treat some cases of early stage cervical cancer in women who want to keep their ability to carry a child, is a radical trachelectomy in which the cervix, upper vagina and tissue surrounding the cervix are removed, but the uterus is preserved. A third option supported by the radiation oncologist was a non-surgical approach – chemoradiation – a combination of chemotherapy and radiation.

Based on the data provided, the team considered the best option for Jem was a radical hysterectomy followed by radiation. The cancer had spread fast and was close to the outer limits of the cervix. But before the decision was made, Michelle called one of her mentors, a retired professor in London, one of the pioneers of the alternative radical trachelectomy procedures, which left the uterus intact. It was clear there were more recurrences of cancer in women who had a treatment of that type. Michelle was certain the recommendation for a radical hysterectomy and radiation was right. But she also knew the impact that would have on her young patient's life. During her fellowship training in gynaecological oncology in Sydney and London, she had learned that, for women, fertility is up there with survival. "There is no easy way to tell a young woman that the treatment she must have to keep her well will also mean she will never bear a child. It takes time to process the implications of treatment that offers long life but which also takes away a life-long dream." As she waited for Jem to arrive, she prepared herself to answer the questions she knew would come: surely there must be another option; what else can I do?

♥   ♥   ♥

In the car travelling to Auckland with her mother and sister, Jem still clung to the hope that the news would be good. She hadn't let her mind go anywhere near what treatment might mean. "Mum's attitude was always that no matter what, we'll deal with that. I was still in that mind frame." Maddy had urged her not to consult Dr Google, but Maddy herself was anxious. She kept repeating the same mantra: we'll be okay. She says, "I thought, I'm 99.9 per cent sure things will be okay, but what if..." Over the previous weeks the sisters had dealt with each new procedure on a case by case basis. "The medical staff avoided 'what ifs'," says Jem. "They don't want to scare you about possible outcomes." The sisters had weathered other traumas in their lives, including the road accident that had claimed a life and severely injured Maddy's best friend, and they were naturally resilient and optimistic. Maddy says, "You never see this at the time, but when you look back there is always a silver lining." Still, she was rocked to the core about events unfolding with her sister. As they walked from the hospital carpark to Michelle's office, she held Jem's hand.

In the waiting room, Jem looked about her. She still couldn't believe this was real. The patients waiting seemed so much older and sicker. Outwardly, Jem was a picture of good health. She thought, 'I shouldn't be here. This is not my place.' I just wanted to be out of there so we could move on with our lives." When they were ushered through, she focused hard on leaving with good news.

Michelle stood up when they came into the consulting room. She held Jem's hand warmly for a moment as Rose and Maddy were introduced. She was pleased there was a support team. "Sometimes the patient is so upset, they can't ask questions or take in information."

Jem remembers thinking Michelle seemed smart and compassionate. "It really felt like she cared." She talked a little about the family. And then she said, "What I've got to tell you isn't good. I'm sorry. But what you need to know is..." Then she drew images of the cervix and the cone biopsy and stepped the three women through the implications of the diagnosis. Rose says she knew immediately Michelle had bad news. "When she began talking about the less important results from the tests, I knew it wasn't good, otherwise she would have told us immediately."

Jem felt the world spinning on its axis. She heard Michelle say the word "urgent" several times. She heard Rose ask whether they could buy some time. "What would happen if Jem became pregnant right away? Could we wait 10 months?" She heard Michelle answer, "Not if you want the baby to have a mother." She knew the specialist had her medical interests at heart and that her only focus was to keep her patient well. "But it was all just shitty to me. I'd never thought of my fertility as tradeable. I'd never thought about being confronted by mortality at 31 years old. Or of thinking I could die. It didn't make sense and it felt too overwhelming to take in."

But then she heard Michelle say, there is another way: you could have a baby a different way and that baby would have two parents. There was a lifeline; slim, but worth grasping by a young woman drowning in grief. Michelle would remove lymph nodes within a week to prevent the cancer spreading further, but she would wait a month before performing the hysterectomy. A month in which Jem could produce eggs that could be harvested to make a baby. It would be tight; it might not work, but it was a glimmer of hope in an otherwise dark tunnel. Michelle said, I suggest you go downstairs to the fertility doctors immediately to see what is possible.

What was possible, it appeared, was precious little. First there were forms to fill in. Do you have a partner? Yes, she wrote. But not a spouse. We've been together only eight months. We're not sure whether he will agree to donate sperm at this stage of the relationship. But we will consider a sperm donor. Beep. Wrong answer. You can't have a donor if you have a partner; you have to work with your partner. But we don't have time, said Jem. The doors seemed to be closing on the small glimmer of hope she had held when she left Michelle's consulting room. She felt desperate and despondent. How could she put pressure on Mark to father their baby at this stage of their relationship? They were in love, but she had no idea what his reaction to fathering her baby would be. She looked at the forms that seemed to suddenly be the barrier to anything she hoped for. "It felt cold and not nice. I was looking for options, but they seemed totally removed from what I was going through." She left the building, again in floods of tears. They seemed to have come to the end of the road.

But she hadn't counted on her mother. "Mum was like a soldier going into battle," she says. While Rose held steadfastly to the view that her daughter's life was more important than any future grandchild, she also knew how desperately Jem wanted a child. "We will get you a baby," she reassured her daughter, searching her brain for solutions. She phoned a friend whose daughter was a GP who had trained with people who were now fertility specialists. She worked out that, because Jem lived in Hamilton, she could deal with a Hamilton-based fertility clinic. Within 30 minutes Rose had made contact with Fertility Associates in Auckland, a private clinic founded in 1987 by two doctors who introduced IVF (Invitro Fertilisation) to New Zealand. It also had a clinic in Hamilton. The waiting list for assessment would normally be six weeks. Rose secured an appointment for her daughter in three days. Jem said the difference in attitude was extraordinary. "They said, 'Jem, whatever you need, we will get you'." It was the first time she had felt optimistic in weeks. She felt re-energised. But she still had to talk to Mark about their options.

Mark was at work on the day of Jem's appointment with Michelle. He knew the news from Auckland was likely to be tough. He had been unable to concentrate while he waited for her call. He felt deeply for the woman who had come into his life a few months before. And he was desperately worried about her health. When she phoned him to ask him to meet her at her mother's home, she was crying as though her heart was broken. They sat in the garden while he tried to come to terms with the news. Jem had a life-threatening disease; she needed to have a major operation within a month to keep her well. His only thought was that he didn't want to lose her. An operation was surely the best option. But her grief was also for the loss of future babies. He held her while she cried, telling her over and over her health was far more important to him than anything else.

Rose and Maddy meanwhile were on another mission to find something that would stem the pain of loss. On the drive home from Auckland, Rose had decided Jem needed a puppy – and she needed it that day. The family had always been dog-lovers. Maddy knew her own dog Wally, had helped her through some tough times. Rose also had a dog. "We wouldn't normally get a puppy without checking with the person, but these weren't normal times," says Maddy. "Jem needed something to distract her and to keep her focused on the moment, not on a future which looked frightening. She needed a fur baby." Again, Rose put her contacts to good use. She phoned the SPCA and scoured Trade Me listings. Then she texted a friend who knew someone with a pet shop. "We have just had a litter of three Maltese Shih Tzu cross puppies come in for sale," she said. It seemed fate was on their side.

When they returned, Jem and Mark were still sitting outside talking. Maddy approached her sister with a clean nappy and blindfolded her. Jem protested, saying she was not in the mood for games. Then she felt a little furry body on her lap, followed by another. For an hour they rolled around on the grass with the pups which had no inkling of the drama unfolding around them. Jem and Mark chose a female and named her Frankie; Rose took one herself and the third pup went to a friend. It had seemed risky at the time, but a counsellor was later to say it was one of the best things they could have done. Animals need you. They keep you in the present, she said.

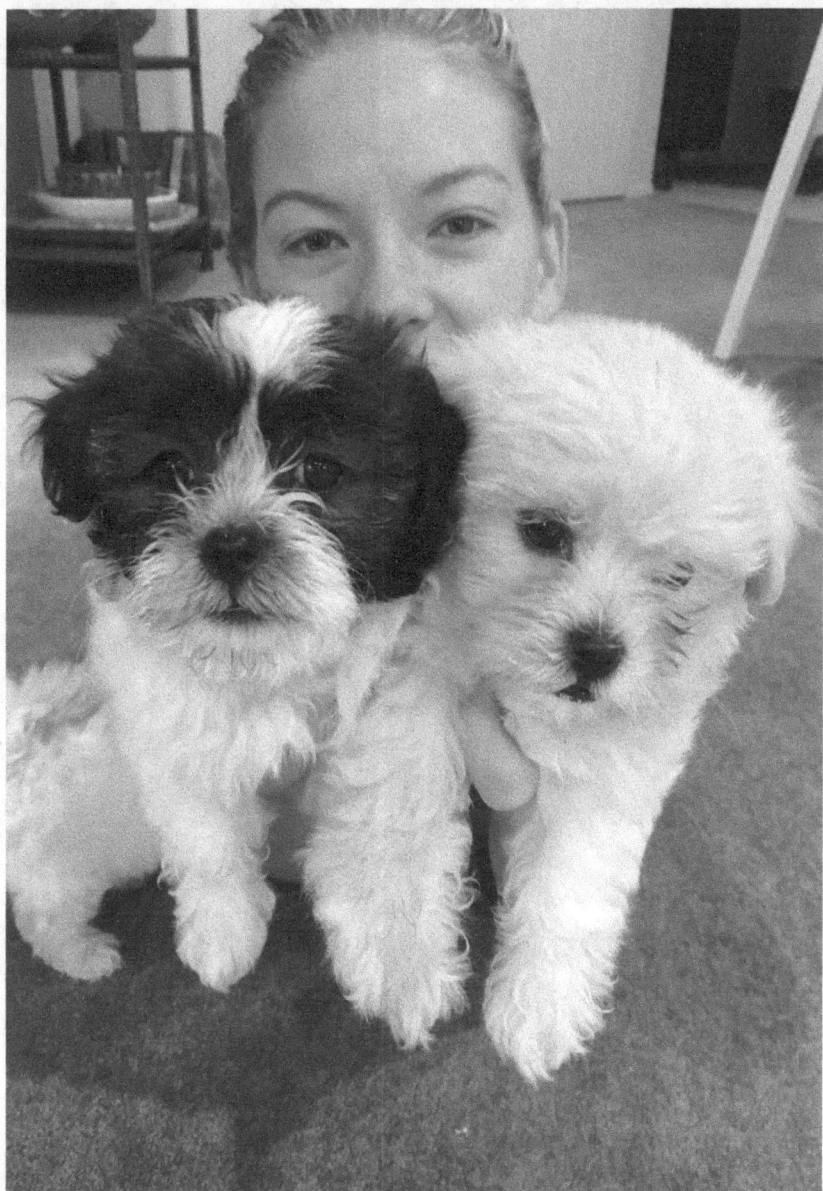

Fur babies help to ease the grief following her
hysterectomy. Jem with Frankie, left and Lulu, her
mother's puppy.

# CHAPTER 4

# A race against time

Jem was now in a race against time. With the deadline for the hysterectomy a month away, and little time to harvest her eggs, she visited Fertility Associates in Hamilton where she was pumped full of GONAL-f, a modified version of the body's own hormone to hyper-stimulate the follicles in her ovaries. Normally, hormone levels would be adjusted over time in response to a woman's tolerance of the treatment. But, in Jem's case, there wasn't time. She injected herself once a day with two hormones – one to suppress her natural cycle to prevent eggs being released before collection; the other to increase the number of eggs produced. The first jab near her tummy button felt like a pin prick; the second like a hot poker had been thrust into her belly. Over the next few weeks, she carried a little chilly bin with her to keep the drugs temperature-controlled.

The hormones caused her ovaries to become swollen and painful. They also made her psychotic. "I'd just rage at my situation and the grief was unbearable. I was totally irrational and a real bitch to be around." Maddy had to steal her phone at times so she wouldn't vent her anger to Mark. She says, "There was no reasoning. These things were just coming out of my mouth with no filter. It was like PMS (pre-menstrual syndrome) on speed." Maddy knew her sister was riding a rollercoaster, and she had to ride it with her. "We've had stressful times before. I know she gets angry but she quickly cools off. When we were kids, she'd react and then think about it and wind back." She also felt for Mark who was seeing his loving partner turn into a harridan. Maddy thought, if Mark hasn't run from all this, he's the one for Jem. Because this is the worst time in the history of her life.

Mark, meanwhile, was struggling with his own demons. He knew Jem wanted him to father their potential child. He also knew there was extraordinarily little time to make a decision. His first son, Ethan, was born when he was just 17 and he didn't learn that he was a father until Ethan was three years old. His first reaction was shock and then disappointment that he had not been told earlier. The experience had made him wary of making decisions about future children. What if he and Jem broke up? What if he fathered a child that could be lost to him? How would parenthood affect their relationship? He and Jem had been together for just eight months. He was establishing a landscaping business, plus his son was now living with him fulltime. He went round and round in his mind. He knew Jem was considering a sperm donor as a back-up option.

Jem was also worried. She knew if Mark was the sole donor and their relationship broke up, he could withdraw his consent. Over the next few days and nights with the clock ticking, the couple talked late into the night, going backwards and forwards over options. Jem understood Mark's hesitation. She knew how affected he had been by the news he had a three-year-old son. But she also needed him to make a decision. Time was running out.

One evening, aware of his son's distress, Mark's father called in unexpectedly. The pair were close and Mark valued his father's views. While Jem was at her mother's house and Ethan out with friends, he and his father had a deep and private conversation. It's not clear exactly what was said, but Mark later told Jem, "I'll do it." No ifs; no buts. Jem was blown away. "Mark was my rock. I thought if we are going to get through all of this in such a pressure cooker situation, I can't see how our relationship won't work."

Seven eggs were harvested by Fertility Associates in Auckland. The procedure would normally have been done vaginally, but because of the risk of transferring cancer cells to the ovaries, it was done laparoscopically. The specialist took care to avoid the scar tissue from previous surgery to remove Jem's lymph nodes. Mark sat in to watch the procedure and witness the first steps towards fathering a child with Jem. He was mesmerised by the science and precision of the process. For the first time it hit home what they were doing. He was also able to report back to Jem what she had said during the procedure. The drugs administered to her were the same ones implicated in the drug overdose of Michael Jackson. Mark told her later, "babe, you were high off your arse."

The same day he donated his sperm and then they sat back to anxiously await the news. Not all fertilised eggs make the grade. But the ones that do are healthier and stronger and more likely to grow into healthy babies. Jem was optimistic, but anxious. As she went about her days, she tried to focus on a future baby taking shape in the lab. Maddy and her mother phoned constantly. No, she said each time. No news yet. She was making a cup of tea when the clinic rang. Five fertilised eggs had survived the five days in a petri dish to blastocyst stage, in which the inner group of cells becomes an embryo. Two embryos were able to be frozen. Jem wept, knowing that she and Mark had done everything in their power to create a baby. As she prepared for the operation that would mean she could no longer carry a child, she held to the thought that there were potential babies waiting to be born.

❤   ❤   ❤

A month after her appointment with Michelle Harris, Jem was admitted to Greenlane Hospital. The view from her window was of Rangitoto Island and the Hauraki Gulf. The island's volcanic cone looked stunning, but she was in no mood to notice. The past few weeks had taken its toll, physically and mentally. There had been so many tests; so many procedures. She was tired and sad. She was also missing Mark, who had left for a long-planned – but ill-timed – trip to visit his brother and family in London. Jem had insisted he go. "He'd been through so much with me. He needed a break."

Rose, Maddy and her daughter Amelia delivered her to her hospital room and then camped in the Cancer Society Lodge across the road from the hospital. As the time neared for her operation, Jem was nervous but reassured by Michelle Harris' approach. "She had this lovely warm, nurturing attitude, but I also knew she was good at her job." In the operating suite, as she drifted into unconsciousness, she let her thoughts drift back to Costa Rica and the image of a new moon.

In a radical hysterectomy the womb, cervix and surrounding tissue are surgically removed. The ovaries may also be removed, but Jem's were left intact, although with no guarantee they would still produce eggs after treatment because of potential damage from radiation treatment that would follow the operation. Radiation is a standard therapy that kills cancer cells through DNA damage. But it can also have an unintended effect of damaging normal tissues within the treatment field. The ovaries are particularly susceptible. Michelle worked hard to find a safe place to rehouse them near the ribs.

The incision for the hysterectomy was made horizontally, which is better cosmetically, but harder for the surgeon, because – unlike a vertical incision, such as for a caesarean section – it cuts through muscle. The transverse cut also made moving the ovaries harder. In the four-hour operation, the pear-sized organ which would normally provide a place for the foetus to grow until birth was taken from Jem's body.

Both surgeon and registrar were pleased with their work. Later, the registrar would tell Jem he was proud of his stitching, which he said would produce only the smallest of scars. But, two days later, complications set in. Jem started projectile vomiting; she couldn't eat and the pain was intense. A perforated bowel was suspected and she was taken back into surgery where the tidy stitches were removed to enable further investigation. Maddy and Rose waited with increasing concern. In London, Mark phoned constantly wanting updates, feeling isolated from what Jem was going through and knowing she was at her lowest ebb.

In fact, the bowel was not perforated, but it had stopped working – not uncommon in young women after a major operation, Michelle Harris says. "While we know this happens and the bowel will return to normal, it's hard for the patient." For Jem, however, it was another huge blow. For two weeks, she was fed through tubes. She felt physically sick, but – as well – the reality of the loss of her uterus hit home. One Friday night, when she was feeling particularly wretched, Michelle stopped by her bed on her way out to dinner. She sat beside Jem and talked about grief. "She knew what she had done, and how that would affect me," Jem says. "She knew I was now healthy, but there are so many other layers."

Rose watched her daughter's struggle with recovery and grief with sadness and concern. She stayed beside her bed, showered with her to wash her hair, and shopped for luxurious nightwear to cheer her up. She also corresponded constantly with Michelle, asking for medical research papers that would increase her knowledge about the disease and treatment. "She (Michelle) always took the time to answer and explain." When Mark returned and rushed to her side, Jem was wraith-like and exhausted. "He was too scared to hug me because I had tubes everywhere. He didn't want to break me. I had to be hooked up to a walking pod. Mum had to get in the shower with me to wash my hair." But her room was filled with bright flowers and gifts from friends and well-wishers. The nurses said it was lovely to enter a room filled with so much love. Mark had also brought gifts from every place he had visited, including an Irish proverb that begins, "May the road rise up to meet you, may the wind be always at your back, may the sun shine warm upon your face..." It seemed a good omen for their future lives together. The couple also gave Michelle Harris a gift of gratitude: a small angel that today she still keeps on her desk.

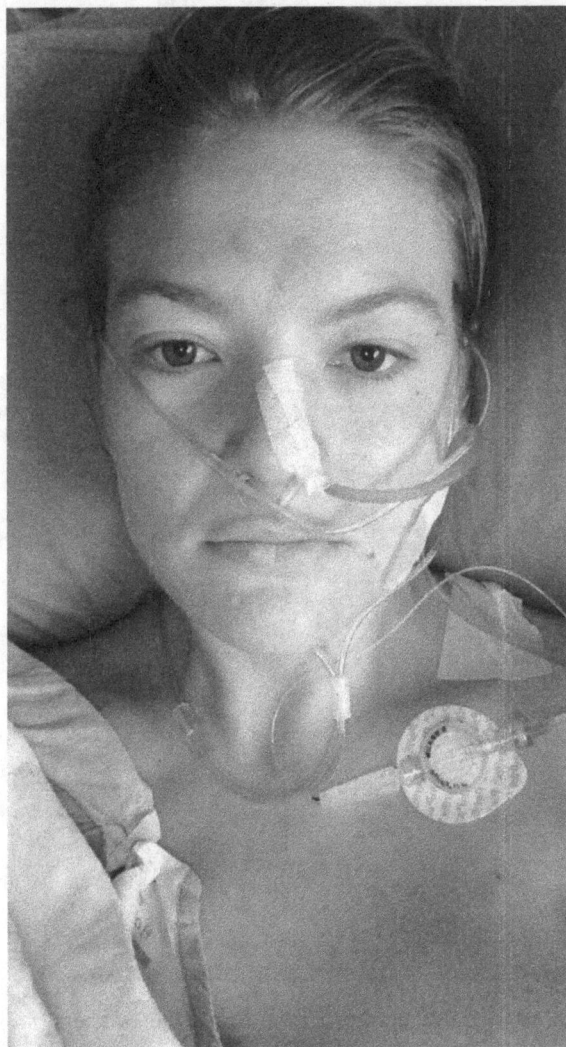

The sad days.
Jem following
her hysterectomy
at Auckland's
Greenlane Hospital.

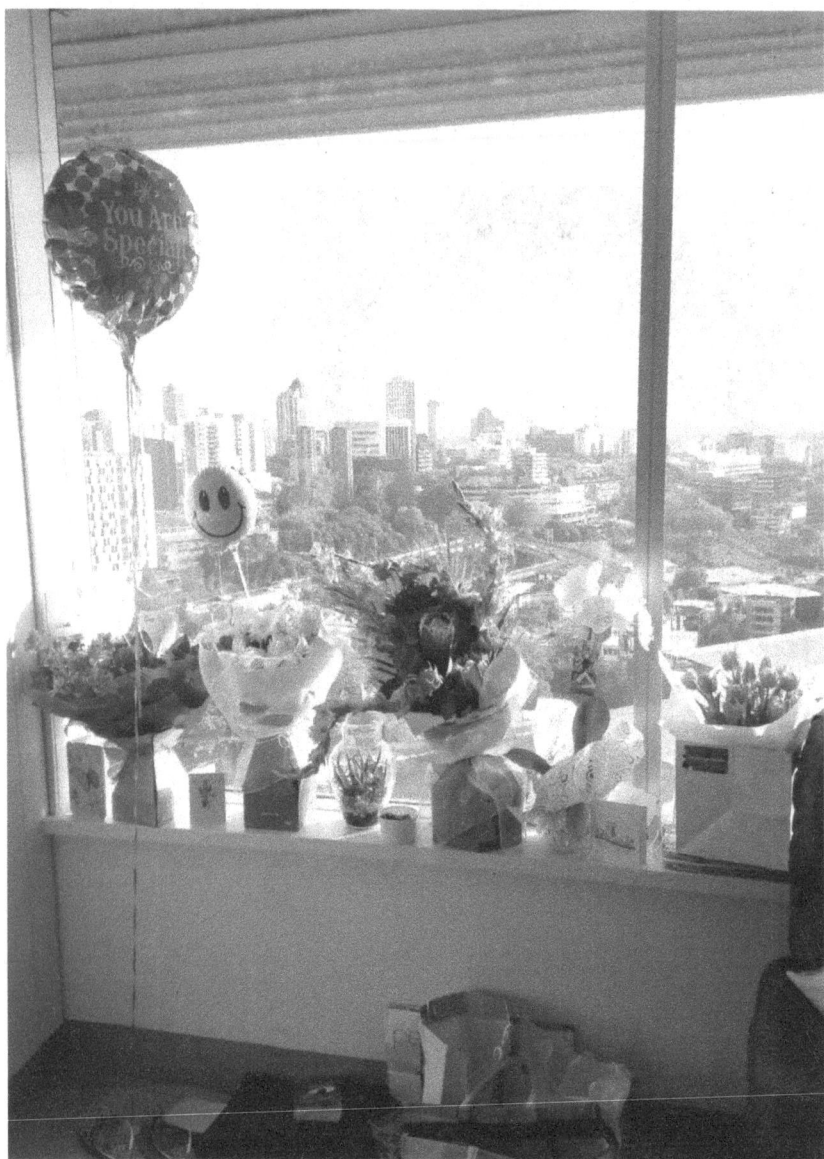

The hospital room was filled with flowers from friends and well-wishers.

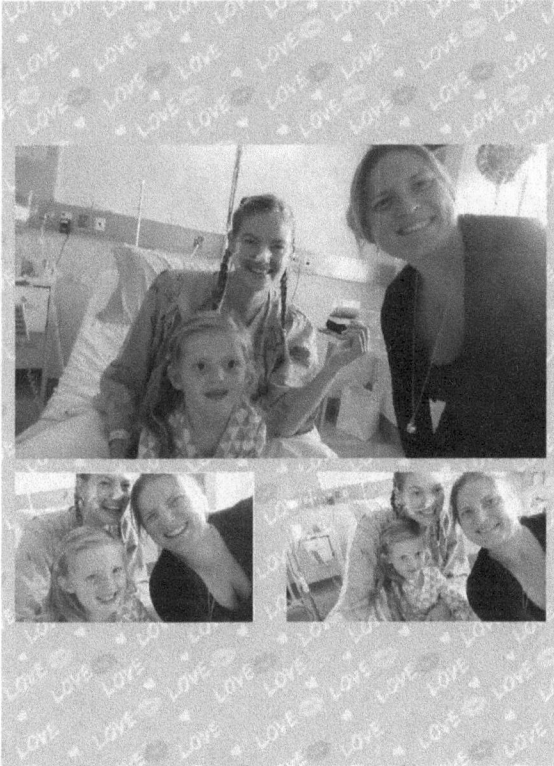

A wraith-like Jem posts a montage of pictures on Facebook when Maddy and her daughter Amelia visit after the operation.

# CHAPTER 5

## the road to recovery

Discharge from hospital should have been a cause for celebration and Jem looked forward to feeling the summer sun on her face and a return to some sense of normalcy. But she was woozy from pain-killers, frail and still in deep grief. Her father insisted she stay with him by the beach at Whitianga to rest and recover. Henry and his wife, Anne, had both had health scares. Henry had had a benign tumour in his pituitary gland below the brain and above the nasal passage; Anne had had breast cancer. They understood the effects of an anaesthetic and the long battle back to health. They wouldn't let her lift a kettle. Because the surgical cut was horizontal, even sitting up was difficult. Jem read, chewing through a book a day "mostly crappy, easy to read ones." She slept a lot and, in the evening, talked to Henry and Anne about her fears and dreams. She had been estranged from her father for several years when she was a teenager after her parents' marriage broke up, blaming him for the separation, and she enjoyed their long chats into the evening. Henry fussed over his daughter, helping her regather her strength. As a counsellor, he tried to paint a positive picture of the future, reassuring her that life would go on, even without children. But she wasn't ready to hear that. "I guess he was trying to prepare me for disappointment. He was trying to be upbeat about it. He was also saying that my health was more important than my fertility. But I don't think he got it. I don't think anyone gets it. I didn't even want to contemplate a life without kids."

When Mark came to pick her up two weeks later, he was pleased to see her looking more like her old self. When he had first seen her in hospital, he had been shocked by her ravaged body. Jem had tried hard not to unload on him while he was in London, so she didn't go into great detail about the complications following her operation. "I just basically said, I feel like shit and everything sucks." Which was how she was feeling.

Back in Hamilton, Mark had been making his own changes. He and Ethan had been living in a rental property in need of renovation, but his parents had bought a property in Hillcrest and suggested he move in. The house was sunny with a garden and room for vehicles for Mark's business. It was an ideal home for Jem to return to, but on the day of the move, she could only watch on the sideline, as Mark's friends hoisted furniture into their new home. While she had stayed over most nights at Mark's former home, she still kept some clothes stashed at her mother's house. They were edging towards their new life as a couple. "The house and our decision to live together seemed like a new beginning. This was really our house. It felt good to have that security."

But there were still further decisions to make. The Greenlane Hospital team had been divided on the need for adjuvant radiotherapy following surgery. On a scale of risk of the cancer returning without radiotherapy, Jem was bang in the middle, making it hard to make a decision. Cervical cancer is a relatively treatable disease and the chances of it recurring are around 35 per cent, usually within two years. Jem felt her body had already been through a lot and resisted the idea of further treatment that could have side effects. Her support team was also divided. Maddy knew her sister was worn out. She was reluctant for her to go through another treatment. Mark was equally adamant she should take every step to ensure the cancer did not return. Jem spent hours researching risks and benefits as they weighed up the pros and cons. She also talked to her surgeon Michelle about how test groups were made up and how ethnicity and age might have a bearing on the results. And she talked to the clinical team's radiation oncologist, Dr Herman van der Vyver. He said bluntly, "You absolutely need this treatment. If you were my daughter, I'd drag you in (for treatment) kicking and screaming." In the end, she made the decision through her own risk assessment. "I thought, if the cancer came back, how would I feel about my choice. I decided if it did return and I had had the treatment, I would know I had done everything within my power to prevent it."

By now, Jem had been discharged from the care of the Auckland DHB and transferred to Waikato Hospital, a five minute drive from the law firm where she worked. It was a relief after the long treks to Auckland but the daily visits over five weeks to the radiation oncology department took their toll. She worked from nine to noon, had the treatment, then went home to sleep. The first day was intimidating. The success of external radiation therapy depends on pinpoint accuracy and Jem lay still as tiny tattoos were marked on her pelvis. She thought of her ovaries tucked out of harm's way beneath her rib cage. While she knew two healthy embryos had already been frozen, she was also optimistic she would still be able to produce eggs after treatment to increase her chances of motherhood if anything went wrong. It was hard to remain positive. "The last week of treatment I felt like I'd been run over by a bus. I had a massive meltdown and said to my boss, Scott, 'I'm just not coping'." She was worried her position at the law firm would be filled by a new graduate. Scott told her to come in only when she felt like it. He also told her he would offer her a fulltime contract when she had completed the treatment.

Jem was grateful that her future employment was secure but getting back into normal life brought its own stresses. Friends, who had followed her illness with concern, showered her with gifts and cards. Every day, she would arrive home to a parcel on the doorstep: hampers of food, therapeutic oils and jewellery appeared. One friend put together a *Book of Fuck, Yeah, You Can Do This,* filled with inspirational quotes and sketches that captured her feelings and reduced her to tears. The same friends wanted her back in their lives to celebrate her wellness. But she wasn't ready. On the night following her final treatment, she and Mark were invited to a friend's 30th birthday. Jem went to Rose's house to have her hair and make-up done and get dressed. But, when Mark came to pick her up, she became anxious and upset. It all seemed too much. "Let's just go for a drink by ourselves, bub," said Mark. They went to a quiet pub until Jem felt ready to try again. But her head wasn't into it. "I didn't feel normal. I was uptight and I didn't want to be around smokers and people living normal lives. I was so sad." After a short time, they left.

Jem worried that Mark would get frustrated. Even though they were living together, she felt anxious he would find the ongoing ups and downs too hard. When she was alone, she still raged and wept. Then she got a letter from the Cancer Society. "It asked if I was feeling down and depressed. It talked about all the things I was experiencing. It was like it had been written by God himself or someone who could read my mind. It posed the questions: where are you going with your life and how are you getting on getting back to normality?" The society asked if she would like to be part of a pilot programme for people who had had cancer. For a young woman, the prospect of group chats with other cancer patients – most of them older – could have been off-putting. But for Jem, struggling with self-doubts and confusion about the future, it came at the right time. She replied 'yes', immediately.

The course had been put together by Cancer Society nurses and a mindfulness coach, based on their understanding of the needs of patients before and after treatment. For many there had been unforeseen side effects, like memory loss and lack of confidence around driving and other routine tasks. Many found it hard to adjust to reality and slot back into their former lives. They told their stories without fear of derision or surprise. Those who were shy in the beginning began to open up as they developed trust in the others. There were tears and laughter and affirmation of the need for positivity. While the group of around 20 were mostly older, their experiences resonated with Jem. One woman of her age had had bowel cancer and had held off treatment until after the birth of her child. Others were isolated from friends and family. "It put things into perspective. It started to make me feel grateful that I had so much support. It was a place where you could say things that you really felt; where you didn't have to hold back to save people's feelings." She started to believe this was a chapter of her life, not the end. At home, she found it easier to open up to Mark and to share her hopes and fears. "I'd come home from the session and try to make sense of the new normal. I'd cry and he would just hold me and stroke my hair. I talked and he listened. I don't know how I could have got through this part without him. He was my true north."

But there were still moments of despair and anger. And she continued to question her own self-worth. "Why would you want to stay with me?" she asked Mark often. One day she felt particularly wretched. When the alarm went off, she lay in bed, refusing to go to work. Mark took the hard line. "Come on, you can't stay in bed all day," he said, pulling her to her feet. He took her to the driving range where they smacked golf balls, until she felt better. They signed up for a mindfulness course. On the advice of her father, Jem kept a diary and became more aware of the triggers that sparked her moods. She talked to the mindfulness coach, who taught her to be aware of her thoughts and how to control them. He pointed out that her shoulders looked as though they were pinned to her ears. "You're trying to hold everything together," he said. She noted things that helped. Going for walks and bike rides was therapeutic; a glass of wine relaxed her. Work was stimulating. She had completed her duty lawyer qualifications and was enjoying the challenge of being in court.

Yet the overwhelming grief of not being able to bear a child was still ever-present. "Every time I'd get a phone call to say someone was pregnant, it would hit me again. Anna was pregnant, Amanda was pregnant, Katie was pregnant, Tracey was pregnant. I'd say, 'That's fantastic', then I'd bawl my eyes out. I was so happy for them, but so jealous and upset for me. That was really tough. There were baby showers and first birthday parties for friends' children. I wanted to be there and be happy for them but it was just a constant reminder that I couldn't have that. That would trigger that insecurity in me. I would think, why would Mark want to be with me when I can't give him that? So I'd be snappy and bitchy, pushing him away." Maddy, watching her sister closely saw what was happening. She knew the cause and she knew the solution. One day she phoned and said, "you know when I told you earlier that you could have my womb to have your baby, you know I meant it, didn't you?" Suddenly, there was a whole new focus. Parenthood was possible. Her sister's offer confirmed that what Jem had dreamt would happen, could come true. Jem, Mark, Maddy and Joe turned their collective thoughts to pregnancy.

CHAPTER 6

# Surrogacy in New Zealand

Surrogacy is not for the faint-hearted. It is a complex and strictly administered process involving health checks, drawn-out applications for approval from various agencies, medical consultations, and hours of counselling for all parties. In New Zealand, while there is no specific surrogacy legislation, there are laws that relate to surrogacy arrangements. One is the Human Assisted Reproductive Technology Act (1994), designed to protect the interests of (particularly) women and children; the other, the Adoption Act (1955), which many argue has no place in today's environment in relation to surrogacy (more about that later). There are also specific criteria around who is eligible. Surrogacy is only approved if a woman has a medical condition that prevents her from becoming pregnant (for example a hysterectomy) or she has unexplained infertility and been unable to become pregnant through other treatments. In New Zealand, it is also illegal to pay surrogates, apart from medical expenses related to the pregnancy, an issue which is also strongly debated. Commercial surrogacy is legal in countries, such as India, Russia and the Ukraine and some states in the US. In California, surrogates can earn around $US40,000 ($NZ61,000). For this reason, some people go abroad to countries where payment is allowed. Others spread the word via social media that they are seeking a surrogate in the hope a stranger will come forward. Despite the hurdles they face, worldwide more couples – including men – are entering surrogacy arrangements and more are being approved. An increase in celebrities such as Kim Kardashian, Elton John, Sarah Jessica Parker, Nicole Kidman, and Olympic diver Tom Daley has raised the profile of surrogacies. In New Zealand, in 2018, 26 applications were received and 20 approved, up from 16 applications and 16 approvals a decade before.

The formal process begins with a doctor's check to determine that surrogacy is the best option for the intending parents. Jem was a clear candidate as she was unable to carry her own child; Maddy had had three full-term pregnancies and completed her family. Each couple then had to take part in three counselling sessions, two separately and one jointly to ensure they had a mutual understanding of the choice they had made. Jem asked to see Sue Saunders, a counsellor at Fertility Associates in Hamilton whom she had first met when she underwent infertility treatment to stimulate egg production before her hysterectomy. She liked Sue's approach and felt confident that she understood her grief and her determination to focus on a future that included a child. Sue had been a counsellor for 36 years – 18 with Fertility Associates in Hamilton – and over that time had seen thousands of couples facing infertility concerns. She had also experienced first-hand the sadness of not being able to conceive. Her first daughter was adopted after six years' trying, and failing, to stay pregnant. When she met Jem and Mark, she noted their love for each other. "Mark said he was determined to see it through to the end. Given what they had been through in the early stage of their relationship with Jem's cancer, I felt confident he would."

Counselling is required by law in surrogate arrangements to ensure couples are fully aware of the legal, emotional, and social implications of their choice. A counsellor's report forms part of the assessment undertaken by ECART (the Ethics Committee on Assisted Reproductive Technology) established under the HART Act, which approves or declines applications. The sessions cover a vast landscape of issues intending parents and intending surrogates and their partners need to get their heads around. Things like the time framework (it takes six months generally to get to the E-CART approval stage, then often three months to get to the implant stage and two years from go to whoa with a successful pregnancy); the potential for disputes between couples; discussions over how the pregnancy is managed by the surrogate – what she eats and drinks; a birth plan; health issues, especially mental health concerns; guardianship of the resulting child and highly sensitive issues such as the storage of embryos (there is a limit of 10 years) plus what happens if an abnormality is detected in the foetus and a decision needs to be made about a termination. But the sessions also cover emotional issues. Sue says the purpose is to ensure couples accept their situation. "When an embryo is made, the couple has to work through the grief of not being able to carry their own baby. They can't control all things. Trust has to be assumed. It's a big thing to go through. Infertility following a cancer diagnosis is a double whammy. When a woman has cancer and finds she is going to have to have her uterus removed, the trauma is huge. Physically she's debilitated; emotionally, her dreams have been whipped away. To even consider IVF when you are looking at your fallibility is a huge thing. Jem had to face all of that and Mark had to face it too. If something were to have happened to Jem, Mark would have had to make a decision about the embryos they had made. We would never offer this option unless there was enough reason to think she would survive."

After the first meeting Jem and Mark also had to apply to Oranga Tamariki – the Ministry for Children – to legally adopt the child from Maddy and Joe, a process now regarded by many as antiquated. Under the Adoption Act, passed in 1955, when a child is born from surrogacy, the surrogate is the child's legal mother and her partner is also a legal parent, irrespective of any biological relationship, until adoption papers have been formally processed, which can take months. As part of the formal adoption process, the surrogate must confirm she doesn't want to keep the baby and the biological father must apply to adopt. The adoption process, which goes through the Family Court, can take months. For Jem and Mark, that would mean any baby conceived by them and biologically their own child, would be Maddy and Joe's legal child until the approval was signed off. If medical intervention were needed in the first weeks of the baby's life, Maddy and Joe's consent would have to be given, even though they were not the child's biological parents.

Surrogacy has been called "the fertility treatment time forgot". While the law governing other fertility treatments has evolved in response to scientific, technological, and social changes, New Zealand surrogacy law has remained fundamentally unaltered for decades. While there is still division about whether a commercial model like that in some US states should be adopted, (the 2004 HART Act bans any payment other than reasonable or necessary expenses incurred for collection and storage of embryos, counselling, ovulation or pregnancy tests and legal advice to "ensure there is no financial incentive to induce vulnerable people into a surrogacy arrangement") there is significant consensus among intended parents, surrogates, some MPs and some within the legal profession over changes to the Adoption Act. Sue Saunders believes the law is a nonsense. "The simple way around it is to make all the associated parties – the biological parents and the surrogate and her partner – the child's guardians from birth and for the surrogate couple to withdraw from guardianship at a suitable time."

But changes are in the wind. In 2020, Labour Minister of Justice Andrew Little acknowledged the Adoption Act was no longer appropriate to deal with the complexities of surrogacy, saying the Law Commission had been asked to undertake a review which could devise a more modern framework that also safeguarded the interests of children. The review is expected to take place by 2022.

For Jem, Maddy, Mark and Joe, the legal processes were complex and frustrating. Both couples had to engage lawyers. There was a lot of detailed information to work through during counselling. Nevertheless, they found working with Sue Saunders helpful and uplifting. "It felt like, 'wow', we're really doing this," Maddy says. Jem says, "Maddy and I had talked about it so much, we knew mostly what we wanted to do and how we would do it." Nevertheless, there were moments she was overcome with emotion. "In our joint counselling session with Maddy and Joe, Sue asked what we would do if anything happened to me and Mark during the pregnancy. Joe just said matter-of-factly, 'Well, we'd keep it (the baby) wouldn't we'?" as though that was a no-brainer. It felt like we were loved and being supported at every turn."

Sue also forewarned the sisters that they would probably face stresses during the pregnancy. "I told them the first three months can be tough because the surrogate mum may be experiencing morning sickness and tiredness, but it's still largely the honeymoon phase when everyone is incredibly positive. The second half of the pregnancy can be tougher, because the surrogate may be very tired and not feeling supported. She may be struggling to manage the house and look after her other kids." The couples didn't know it then, but that is exactly what would happen.

Sue also talked directly to the men about their feelings. "Men will often be the stable force, while women get caught up in emotion. But they are often feeling overwhelmed. The intending father might not know how to physically touch a woman who is carrying his baby. He may not want to be at the 'business end' during the birth. The surrogate's partner may experience an emotional or sexual difference, knowing she is carrying someone else's child."

While those issues were explored during their counselling sessions, Sue always felt confident the couples were well up to the responsibilities ahead. She sent off the application to ECART with optimism, knowing Jem, Mark, Maddy and Joe and their families were well prepared for whatever lay ahead. While it was not her role to recommend an application went ahead, she knew from all the evidence she had presented ECART would know she was comfortable with them pushing ahead with their plans. Four weeks later, she was advised the application was successful.

# CHAPTER 7

# "I never doubted we would have a baby"

When Maddy texted Jem to say, "you can have my womb", she already had a plan in mind. She wanted to have a year at home with her third child, Harry, and to continue to breastfeed him for that time. She had thought she would then return to work to supplement the family income, but the costs of childcare for her two pre-schoolers made that proposition uneconomical. It made sense to instead focus on a pregnancy for Mark and Jem.

The couples met to discuss dates. Jem was over the moon. "It was like flicking a switch; turning off the grief and turning on the optimism. I thought, 'oh, shit, this can really happen.' I never doubted it would work. Whenever Maddy has become pregnant, she has always had a full-term baby. Perhaps I was naive. But I never doubted she would have our child." Joe was also keen to get on with things and for Maddy to stop breastfeeding Harry, who was 15 months old, and still waking regularly in the night. Amelia had weaned at that age; Lachie had weaned earlier when Maddy returned to work. Maddy resolved to stop breastfeeding before a planned camping holiday in early February. Harry had different ideas. "He really fought me on it," Maddy smiles. "I remember I hadn't fed him for two nights and he wouldn't go to sleep. We were all exhausted." On February 6, Waitangi Day in New Zealand, she looked Harry in the eye and said, "okay, last boob, we're done." And so it was.

Hormone treatment to prepare for the implantation was scheduled for a fortnight later. Maddy worried that it was too soon after weaning Harry. "I remember thinking, 'we need those breast-feeding hormones to be out. I'd only just dried up.'" But she was reassured by the medical staff. For the first stage of treatment, she took prolactin, to inhibit her own ovulation, followed by progesterone and oestrogen to prepare her uterus to support the implanted embryo. An alternative to manufactured ovulation was for her to rely on her own natural menstrual cycle to pinpoint the optimum time for the implant. Medical trials show that there is no difference in the success rates of embryo transplants for natural and HRT (hormone replacement therapy), but the artificial preparation of the lining of the uterus provides options for individual patients and allows clinicians to keep variables under control. For Maddy there were also practical issues to consider. The natural cycle option would have involved daily early morning blood tests for at least two weeks, meaning trips through rush-hour traffic into Hamilton, plus disruptions to family life. She talked to Joe and Jem and Mark. "We thought because it was medicalised it would be far more accurate, plus it gave us some flexibility." Jem was concerned about any potential side effects of the hormonal treatment on her sister, including tiredness, but thrilled they were finally underway.

In the end, Maddy suffered no adverse effects. She was, however, pleased to stop dealing with "pretty yucky pessaries and pills the size of horse tablets'. "They were really hard to swallow, plus I had to remember to take them at a precise time every day." After 14 days, her blood tests were done and implantation was scheduled for three days' time.

On March 15, 2018, Maddy, Jem and Mark arrived at Fertility Associates Clinic in the centre of Hamilton. By now the building had become familiar and staff greeted them by name. They knew how important the day was to couples trying to conceive. Joe was working, so Mark carried Harry, enjoying holding the toddler with whom he and Jem had formed a close bond. Jem was excited. It was the first sight she and Mark would have of their potential son or daughter. Maddy was also pleased to be at the start of what could be a dream outcome for her sister. But she was physically uncomfortable. For the ultrasound that would track the transfer of the embryo, she had to have a full bladder and she was desperate to go to the loo. She hoped the procedure wouldn't take long.

Undergoing IVF is a peculiar experience. In many respects it feels surreal. The moment of conception is usually a mysterious event that takes place in private. With IVF it is a public affair, watched by an audience. The group was shown to the procedure room where Maddy was gowned and prepped. A small hole in the wall, like a 1970s serving hatch, provided a link to the embryology lab, where Embryo No 1 had been stored in liquid nitrogen at -196 Degrees C for 24 months. Thawing to body temperature had begun 40 minutes before. The embryo had been loaded into a delivery tube that would then be inserted into a catheter through Maddy's cervix to her uterus. As the tube was passed through the hatch and the tube was inserted into the catheter, Mark joked, "Are you sure they've got the right one?" Jem watched the screen on the wall monitor. As the tube reached her sister's uterus, the embryo was pushed through into its potential cocoon for the next nine months. There was a white flashing dot, an air bubble that dropped with the embryo, "like a sparkling star", said Jem. She said a small prayer. "Please let this work." Breaths were released and tears shed. Mark stretched his back, aching from holding Harry. Maddy looked for the toilet sign. "It certainly was a very different experience from normal impregnation," she says. "Not at all romantic." The procedure had taken only a few minutes, but it felt like a lifetime. The nurse, who was also pregnant, congratulated them. Jem thought that was a good sign. "There was lots of good baby juju in that room." The group had celebratory breakfast at a café and then headed their separate ways. "Just carry on as normal," was the advice. Jem returned to work at the law firm and Maddy went home to put up her feet for a short time before the older children came home from school and nursery.

Ten days later, Maddy had a blood test. The family gathered at her home to wait for the phone call. Rose had popped a bottle of champagne in the boot of the car in case there was cause for celebration. But the call didn't come. Maddy left with the children to go to a friend's birthday party, Rose also left and Mark and Joe were outside, building a children's playground when Jem's phone rang. She collapsed on the grass, screaming, "We're pregnant," and then rang the others with the news. The champagne – appropriately named G H Mumm – was popped. Jem thought the name was propitious. She poured a small glass – it was to be her last alcohol to support her sister's sacrifices during the pregnancy. It tasted so sweet. She and Mark left on a high and started making plans for their baby.

The following day, Maddy went to an Ed Sheeran concert in Auckland. She had been looking forward to it and she felt buoyed by the previous day's news. The concert lived up to its billing, but during a trip to the loo, she noticed light spots of blood on her pants. It was 11 days after the embryo transplant. "Normally, you wouldn't know you were pregnant. You'd just think it was your period starting." Her heart missed a beat and the remainder of the concert was a blur. The next day she visited her doctor, who confirmed her hormone levels were not at the level they would expect for a pregnancy at that stage. She phoned her sister to prepare her. Three days later she began bleeding heavily. The bleeding lasted for 10 days, double her normal period. A miscarriage was confirmed.

Jem was at work when Maddy phoned. She had been anxious after her sister's call three days before, but still hopeful. The second call rocked her world. "Mark came to pick me up. I was sobbing. I kept thinking, 'why does it have to be so hard for me?' I'd thought pregnancy was so easy for Maddy, so when the blood test confirmed it, I'd assumed we were having a baby. I had never considered another outcome. I had close friends I'd shared the news with. I knew I would have to tell them so as to avoid those awkward moments when they would ask how the pregnancy was going. I was absolutely shattered."

Maddy was also desperately sad and wondered if she had contributed in any way to the miscarriage. "I kept asking myself, 'did I do something wrong? I went backwards and forwards over the past 10 days. I always felt the treatment had begun too soon after weaning Harry. I'd gone from being pregnant and feeding him for over a year to taking hormones for pregnancy. With all these different hormones that come with each part of the process, my body didn't know which way was up. To go straight into hormone treatment 20 days after finishing breastfeeding felt like too soon." She is angry that women's minds immediately go to self-blame. "What did I do wrong? Have I caused this? Women should share what they go through when they miscarry. It is so common and yet people expect we will get over it and move on with our lives. Women need so much support at this time."

Jem and Mark were going through their own nightmare. They had only one viable embryo left. There was no guarantee that Jem could continue to produce eggs. "That one embryo was so precious," Jem says. "But it suddenly seemed precarious."

Maddy also wrestled with some big questions. She knew she had to return to work at some stage, "because we were really broke", but she also didn't want to revoke her offer to Jem and Mark. "The whole point of doing it (the procedure) quickly was so I could return to work in the quickest time. If the next embryo wasn't viable, we would have to wait three months to harvest more eggs from Jem, which would push any further treatment and pregnancy out to the middle of the following year. I thought, 'where do we draw the line?'

For a time the couples remained in shock, assessing what had happened and their options for the future. Jem continued to work but was stressed. Her boss was sympathetic, knowing how much this meant to her. He had supported her through her cancer treatment and felt huge compassion for the young and talented lawyer whose future hopes of carrying a baby had been dashed by illness two years before. The young couples discussed their options separately and at each other's homes. They agreed there was one option: they would try again as quickly as possible with the one remaining embryo. For Maddy, it was the right decision, but the thought of another round of hormone treatments was daunting and at odds with her views about healthy living. Then Joe said, "Why would you take them (the hormones)? You get pregnant if you sneeze." They decided to do it the natural way.

In April, a month after the miscarriage, Maddy returned to work to cover for a colleague who had had a car accident. On her last day at work, she had a blood test to make sure her HCG levels (Human chorionic gonadotropin - a pregnancy hormone produced by the placenta once an embryo implants in the uterus) were back to normal. At the beginning of May, after one more menstrual cycle (her cycles lasted around 36 days), she made the first of 22 half-hour daily treks in to Hamilton from her home at Horotiu to have her blood tests. Her arms were like pin cushions. "It was a bitch," is all she says. Jem, meanwhile, would make the trek in the other direction to Maddy's home to drop the children to school and day-care, before heading to work herself. One day, Maddy had a call from the clinic. "You're about to ovulate, so no shenanigans with your husband," they warned. "You could become pregnant with two babies." Maddy blanched at the idea. "I did not want to be carrying cousins."

In the wider scheme of things, no sex was a small price to pay. Three days later, they returned to Fertility Associates for the second implantation – the last of the embryos made its way into Maddy's womb.

Within four days, she knew she was pregnant. "It felt totally different from the time before. I just knew. I had a feeling of fullness and little cramps; I was tearful and my boobs hurt. I was hormonal." The couples had opted not to have another 10-day test after their previous experience, deciding they would prefer to wait longer in the hope the pregnancy would last. But after 12 days, Maddy snuck out to get a home pregnancy test kit. When she peed on the stick and saw two lines appear, she let out a whoop. She phoned Jem, "Even though we agreed that we were not going to do an early blood test, I am totally pregnant."

At home, Jem let herself dare to belief that this time was different. "I thought, this time. It has to work this time because it is our last embryo. It had to be. Mark was more cautious because he didn't want me to be upset again. But because we had had a different approach without hormonal treatment, I was hugely optimistic and positive. I had convinced myself the first miscarriage was the hormones' fault. I had to reframe it." Maddy says her sister is a hugely positive person. Jem says, "I believe you can't put out too much doubt because what you put out affects what happens. I try not to bring the negative in; I try to fight with it rather than against it." She knew she couldn't put Maddy and Joe in a situation where it could take months longer to harvest new eggs, even if that was possible. "I wanted to move on past the tests and procedures. I thought, this one is different."

And it was. The pregnancy was confirmed.

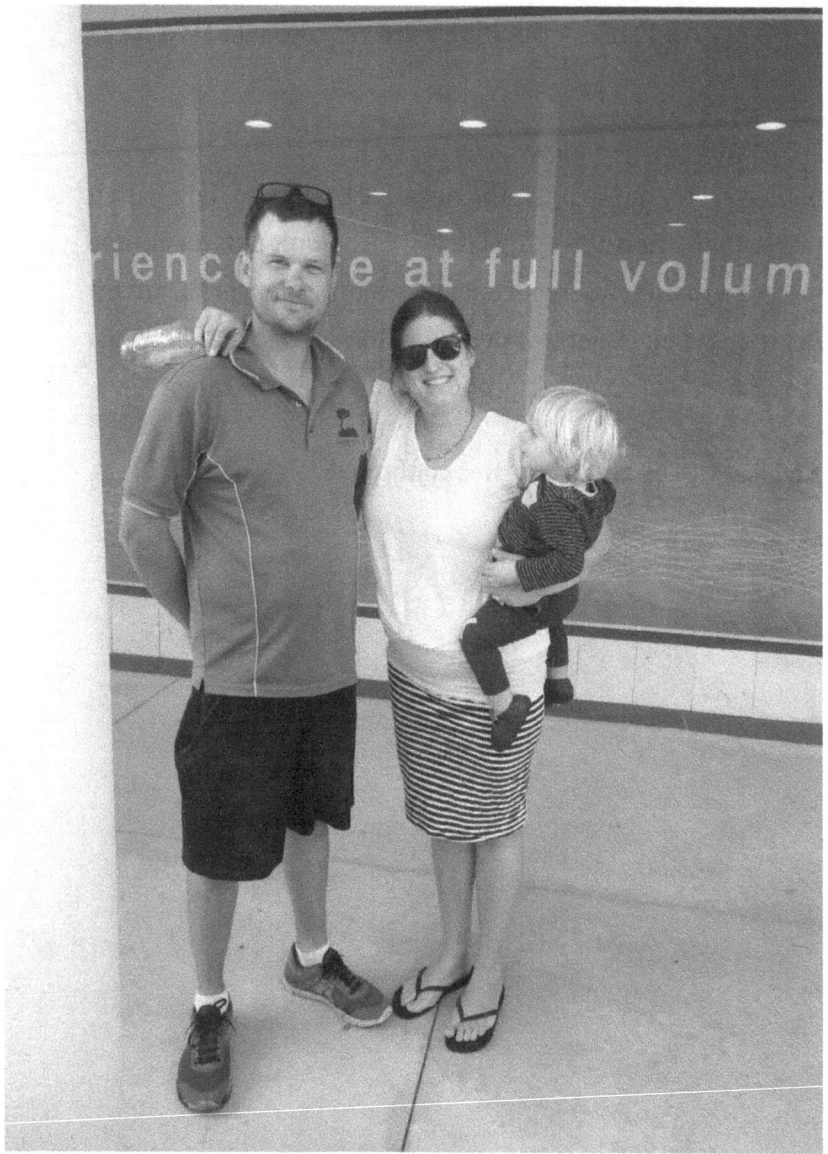

T-Day. Mark with Maddy and Harry, her youngest son,
on the day of the embryo transfer.

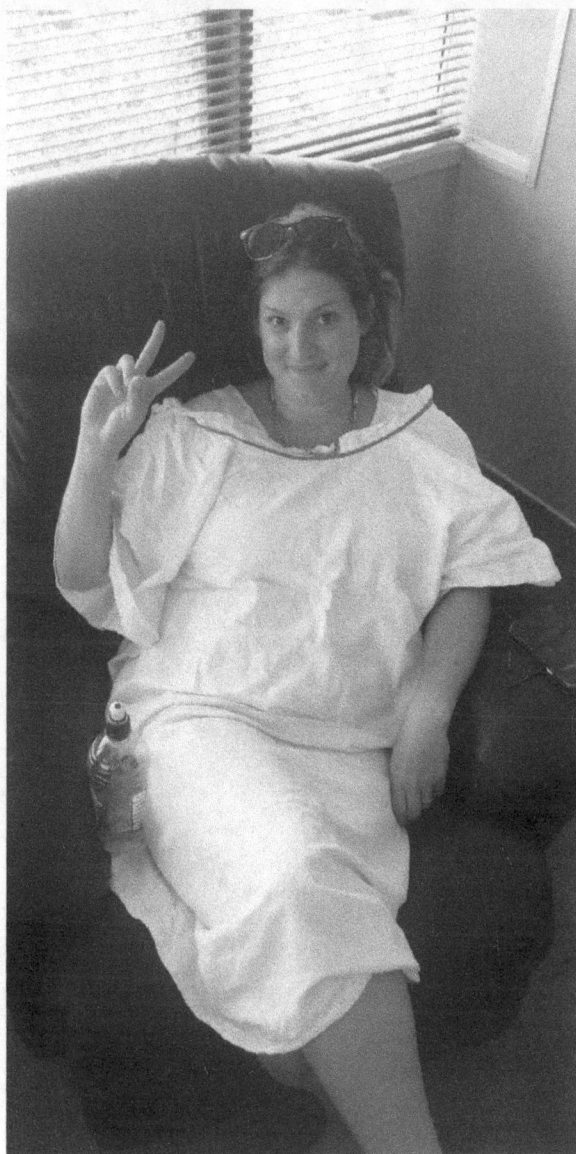

Maddy gives the V for victory sign after the embryo transfer at Fertility Associates clinic in Hamilton.

# CHAPTER 8

# 'You have to keep talking'

If Maddy felt daunted by the prospect of another pregnancy while parenting three young children, to begin with she kept it hidden. But the day after the implantation, Joe left to work in Balclutha in the South Island for six months. He often worked away from home and Maddy had got used to being a sole parent during his absences. Because she seemed well, with no sign of the severe morning sickness she had had with Harry, family, and friends – including Mark and Jem – thought she was doing well. But the exhaustion was intense and Harry, who was 18 months, was still waking often through the night. It was also the start of the winter sport season and the older children had to be transported to their Saturday games. "It was cold and wet. I did not want to take three kids to school sports. Normally, if Joe was home he would do that. You forget that pregnancy sucks you dry. I'd also been told that in a surrogacy your body can detect different genetics, which can make symptoms worse. I was so tired."

She resisted asking for help, knowing Jem was back working fulltime and Rose was away a lot. But she was getting near breaking point. "I couldn't bring myself to clean the shower or cupboards; I was feeding the kids, but I wasn't cooking nutritious meals for myself." She felt alone and physically exhausted. "I just wanted someone to take the children away so I could have a break." When the pregnancy was confirmed, she and Jem had made a pact that Jem would not eat the food that Maddy could not eat during pregnancy, or drink alcohol. One morning, after a rugged night with Harry, Maddy received a snapchat image of Jem in bed eating MacDonald's, watching Netflicks and clearly hungover. It seemed like the ultimate betrayal. She snapped. "I thought, 'You bitch, why are you still in bed. I've been up since 4.30'." She phoned Joe crying, saying 'I'm going to kill one of our children'." He told her to phone Jem to let her know how she was feeling. "She should just know," Maddy cried. Jem says it took the menfolk to bang their heads together and get them to talk to each other, rather than venting.

On Joe's next visit home, the couples held an urgent roundtable meeting about how Maddy was feeling. Jem says it was complete naivety on her and Mark's part. "We didn't know what it was like to have three kids while your husband is away, let alone when you are growing another human for someone else and how exhausting that was. Maddy said she loved that we came out regularly and brought coffee and flowers, but she didn't need that. What she needed was practical hands-on help with the kids and housework." Jem immediately quit her job at the law firm and began working part time for Rose, which gave her more flexibility. She picked up the kids from school and stayed to help with bath times and bed. She and Mark organised food bag deliveries and Jem cooked them for her sister. They also organised a cleaner. The regulations around payment to surrogates are strict but allow for items related to the pregnancy. Both women felt the support came within the guidelines. They say surrogates and parents need to be open with each other and share their feelings. But they acknowledge it isn't always easy. Their relationship had been tested. Jem said, "We're sisters and we can say things and they will be quickly forgotten But if the surrogate is someone you don't know well, that could be different." She knew the surrogacy would never affect their close relationship, but she had other fears that she expressed to Rose. "I thought if the second implantation didn't work, it will be so hard on Maddy."

But Rose says she was never worried her daughters would not be able to sort out any issues arising from a pregnancy. "Our way of dealing with differences as a family is to air them, have a laugh, then a wine, and move on. Dad lived by the maxim 'least said, soonest mended,' which I agree with." She says her daughters have different personalities, but they are always in each other's corner. "Jem is vivacious, a people person; people gravitate towards her. Maddy is quieter; she is kind and generous and she has an equanimous nature. When bad things happen, people turn to Maddy, because she is so even-keeled." Rose had, however, been privately concerned for Maddy's wellbeing during the pregnancy. She had raised four children and knew how tiring a pregnancy could be.

Over the next few weeks the sisters watched in awe as Maddy's belly swelled. Jem and Mark debated whether they wanted to know the baby's sex. Jem was keen, but Mark wanted it to be a surprise. Then a friend, whose partner was pregnant, learned his forthcoming baby was a girl. Mark suddenly realised how special that was. It was a way of connecting with his baby. While Maddy was relaxed about the parents feeling the baby's kicks and patting her belly, to Mark the pregnancy still seemed one step removed. Fertility Associates counsellor Sue Saunders also thought it would help the couple have a closer connection with their baby. At the 20-week scan, the nurse said, "Do you want to know the sex?" When they nodded, she said "You are having a girl." Jem, who had secretly longed to have a daughter, wept with joy in Mark's arms. She had a premonition it would be a girl. "When Maddy was pregnant with Amelia, she craved carrots. Couldn't get enough of them. It's a wonder Amelia wasn't born orange. It was the same with this pregnancy. She always had carrots with her."

The soon-to-be parents pored over the image on the screen of the tiny image of their daughter while Maddy, who had again drunk up large before the scan, urged them to hurry so she could visit the toilet. The first picture of their daughter was stuck on the fridge. They chose the names Grace Madeleine, after the woman who was to bring their baby into the world.

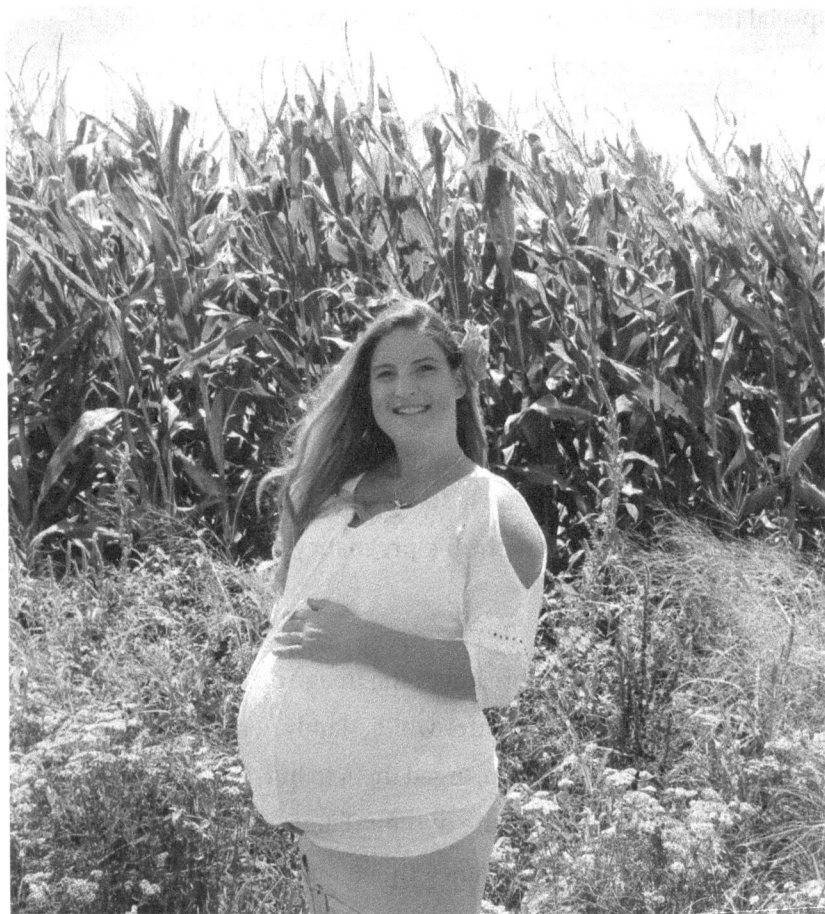

Happiness is a round belly. Maddy treasures the final weeks of her pregnancy.

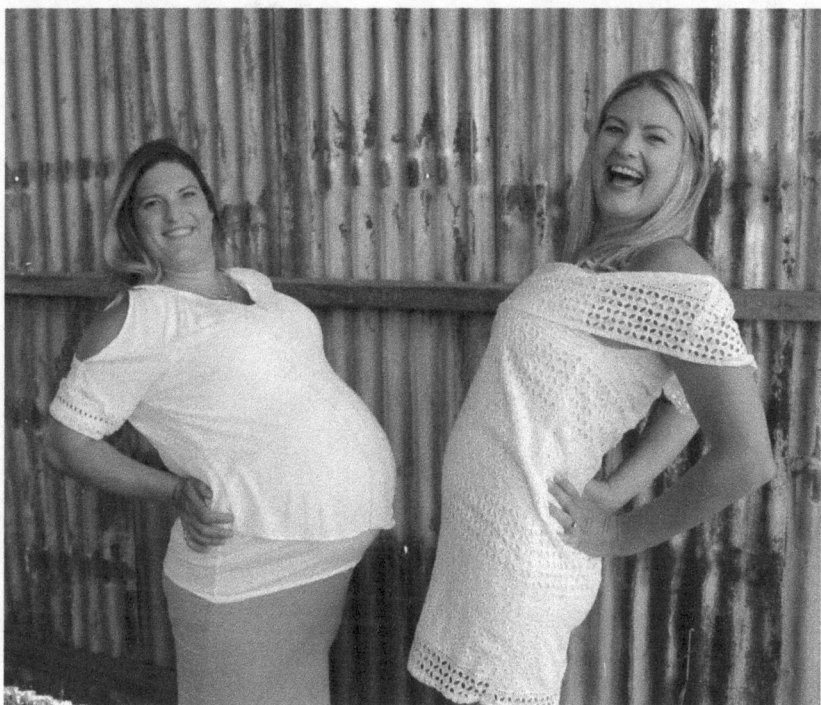

Jem and Maddy. "The greatest good is what we do for one another,"
– Mother Teresa.

# CHAPTER 9

# Yes, you can breastfeed

While Maddy was counting down the months of the pregnancy, Jem was focused on her own project: to establish breastfeeding. She had watched Maddy and her friends breastfeed their babies and still remembered Rose feeding her younger siblings when she was growing up. "Breastfeeding was just part of our family life." Maddy knew of women who had breastfed their babies born through surrogacy and she encouraged Jem to consider it. For Jem, the prospect of feeding the baby she had been unable to bear was exciting, but daunting. "I kept thinking, 'What if I fail? It will just be another thing my body hasn't been able to do. The sadness that could come from failure, knowing breast is best, would be just more pain." Maddy's view was pragmatic: If you can't do it, you don't lose anything, because you can always bottle feed. You're not going to lose anything through trying.

The subject came up when they began meeting midwife Karene to discuss the birth plan. She was hugely supportive and gave Jem a book on the subject and a list of resources to explore. Jem dived into them, wanting to understand the practicalities and the chances of success. "It totally made sense. If you think back to ancient times and in tribal communities, women often fed babies they hadn't borne. In some **traditional cultures, the** baby's grandmother induced lactation routinely in case the mother had problems. Women feeding each other's children was a way of survival." Further inspiration came during a random conversation with a colleague at court. The woman showed her a photo on Facebook of a friend feeding the baby she hadn't birthed. Jem thought, 'if she can do it, so can I'." She had no idea how much it would test her resilience over the next few months.

For a pregnant woman, the production of breast milk is a natural process that occurs through the interaction of hormones and physical changes to the body. During pregnancy, increased amounts of progesterone, oestrogen, and prolactin are produced, readying the breasts for breastfeeding. When the baby is born, prolactin rises and oestrogen and progesterone decrease, which triggers lactation. At that point, the principle of supply and demand takes over: the more the baby feeds and needs, the more milk is produced. During suckling, oxytocin is released, which causes the milk to flow. As these processes occur naturally, a pregnant woman usually needs do nothing until her milk "comes in" at the end of the pregnancy. For women who aren't pregnant, milk production is more complicated, but is entirely possible with medical management. Essentially, the process involves tricking the body into thinking it is pregnant by introducing the same hormones that would naturally occur during pregnancy – progesterone and oestrogen – and the drug Domperidone (a medication more commonly prescribed as an anti-nausea and gastric reflux drug), which, while not a hormone, has the side effect of increasing milk production. The progesterone and oestrogen are administered in the form of a birth control pill to be taken non-stop, skipping the week of placebos, from around five months into the pregnancy. The birth control pill actually suppresses milk supply, mimicking what happens during pregnancy.

On the advice of Karene, Jem opted to follow the guidance of Canadian paediatrician Dr Jack Newman, renowned as a proponent of breastfeeding for mothers who have not birthed their babies. He recommends a series of protocols which cover the timing, dosage of hormones and medication, and pumping.

But, because Jem had had cancer, she was worried. "I was concerned that because I'd had cervical cancer – "a womanly cancer" – and the treatment involved taking female hormones, that that might mean I was susceptible to breast cancer." Mark was also concerned she might be putting herself at further risk. She made an appointment with a female GP and went in armed with print-outs of research and the advice and information she was following. The GP, herself a breastfeeding mother, was reassuring, but also contacted Jem's oncology team in Auckland. They wrote to her saying it was fine to proceed. Cervical metastasis to the breast is considered rare. With health concerns allayed, Jem talked to Mark about what it would involve. "He echoed what Maddy said, 'If you think you can do it babe, just do it'. She knew now she was on a course to do something pro-active and positive for her baby. "I had always admired breastfeeding mums. We grew up in a household where breastfeeding was a natural part of parenting. I'd seen all my friends' boobs. Once it was dangled in front of me that it was possible, I really, really wanted to do it."

Mark marvelled at his partner's commitment. The woman he had fallen deeply in love with had been through so much, but she was determined to do everything in her power to give their child the best start in life. In October, they travelled to Melbourne for a friend's wedding and a much-needed break from the intensity of the past few years. On a day trip to Sorrento Beach, 95km south of the city, Jem kicked off her sandals and paddled in the sea. Mark urged her to take off the ring she wore on her right hand – a precious heirloom from her grandmother – so he could pocket it for safekeeping. When her back was turned, he dropped down on one knee. "Jem, will you marry me?" Then he slipped the ring back on her left hand. Her scream of joy rivalled the cries of the gulls. Mark said later, "I hadn't planned on the location, but it just seemed right." He had phoned Henry and Rose in advance to get their blessing. They returned to New Zealand with new focus: there was not only a baby to plan for, but also a wedding.

On their return from Melbourne, Jem resumed her focus on establishing breastmilk. Just before they had travelled to Australia, she had begun taking a low-level progesterone contraceptive pill. It seemed ironic that pills designed to ensure a woman didn't conceive were now being used to trick her body into thinking it was pregnant. "I've taken contraceptive pills for half my life, but I didn't actually know how they work." At Christmas, three months before the baby's due date, she stopped taking the contraceptive pill and began the course of Domperidone. Her breasts swelled impressively. She also bought a top-end double breast pump (the "biggest, baddest pump I could find"), and began pumping three times a day. Mothers who have pumped to boost or supplement their milk supply know how tiredness, technique and the insatiable appetite of a growing baby can weaken the will to persevere with pumping. But Jem now had a goal in sight. "Once I started doing it (pumping), I was totally committed. If I slipped off the pace, I had Maddy and Karene cracking the whip. Because the baby was growing and pressing on Maddy's bladder, she had to get up in the night to go to the loo. She said to me, 'you should be doing the same thing. Breastfeeding isn't a 9-5 job'."

Pushing aside any thoughts that her sister simply wanted her to suffer with sleepless nights, Jem set her alarm and began pumping through the night. Sessions doubled to six to eight times during 24 hours, with at least one at 2am. She would slip quietly out of bed, trying not to wake Mark, and go through to the nursery already prepared for their baby's arrival. Karene had suggested it would be helpful to pump where she could visualise feeding her baby. It was a positive reinforcement of what she had committed to do. During the day, she rushed home at lunch time, stripped off her corporate jacket and hitched on the pump. "I had my robo-bra on. I looked like a Fembot from Austin Powers (female characters who fought with guns hidden in their large breasts). Robo-boobs." The pump was expensive, but effective. It was electric, but also battery-powered, which meant she could pump while walking around the house.

After pumping for about 4-5 weeks, she was in the shower hand-expressing her breasts when she noticed a small trickle of liquid coming from her nipple. She let out a whoop of excitement. "Got milk," she screamed out to Mark. It was a turning point. "I was ecstatic. As soon as I got that little dribble it was really motivating. I'd get up every night because I knew it was working.

Dr Newman is cautious about the volume of milk women can achieve under the protocols but reassures women that any milk they produce for their baby will be beneficial. Lactation consultants also know that a pump is never as good as a baby that is suckling well and well latched on. At first Jem expressed barely 5mls that would barely wet the bottom of the pump. Then it increased almost daily. In February, the month her baby was due to be born, she was expressing up to 100mls. Each batch was transferred to tiny zip lock bags, labelled, and put into the freezer. On days when she was feeling disheartened, she would look in the freezer and see the mounting piles of bags. On the side line, her cheerleaders, Mark, Maddy and Karene, gave her encouragement. "Karene was amazing," she says. "She never pressured me, but she said, if you want to do it, I'll give you all my support."

Two weeks before the baby was due, Mark and Jem went on a glamping babymoon on a remote farm in the Bay of Plenty. The location was idyllic, surrounded by bush with lanterns to light their way. But no power. Jem knew she had to continue pumping without a break. "I thought, 'no problem', I'll just go on battery power." But the battery wasn't strong enough to create suction. So the couple tramped down the hill to an old farm shed. In the midst of a luxurious weekend away, camped under the stars, Jem hooked herself up to the shed's power supply in what appeared to be the tearoom and pumped, hoping the farmer wouldn't walk past. "The sad thing was I had to tip it out when I'd finished, because there was nowhere to store it."

As the date for the birth drew closer, she felt tired but triumphant, knowing she had done all she could to prepare herself to feed her baby. "I had never understood how hard it was for some women to breastfeed. I just thought your boobs fill up with milk and you do it." She knew what she had done was one of the hardest things she had ever done. But she still didn't know whether she would be able to successfully breastfeed.

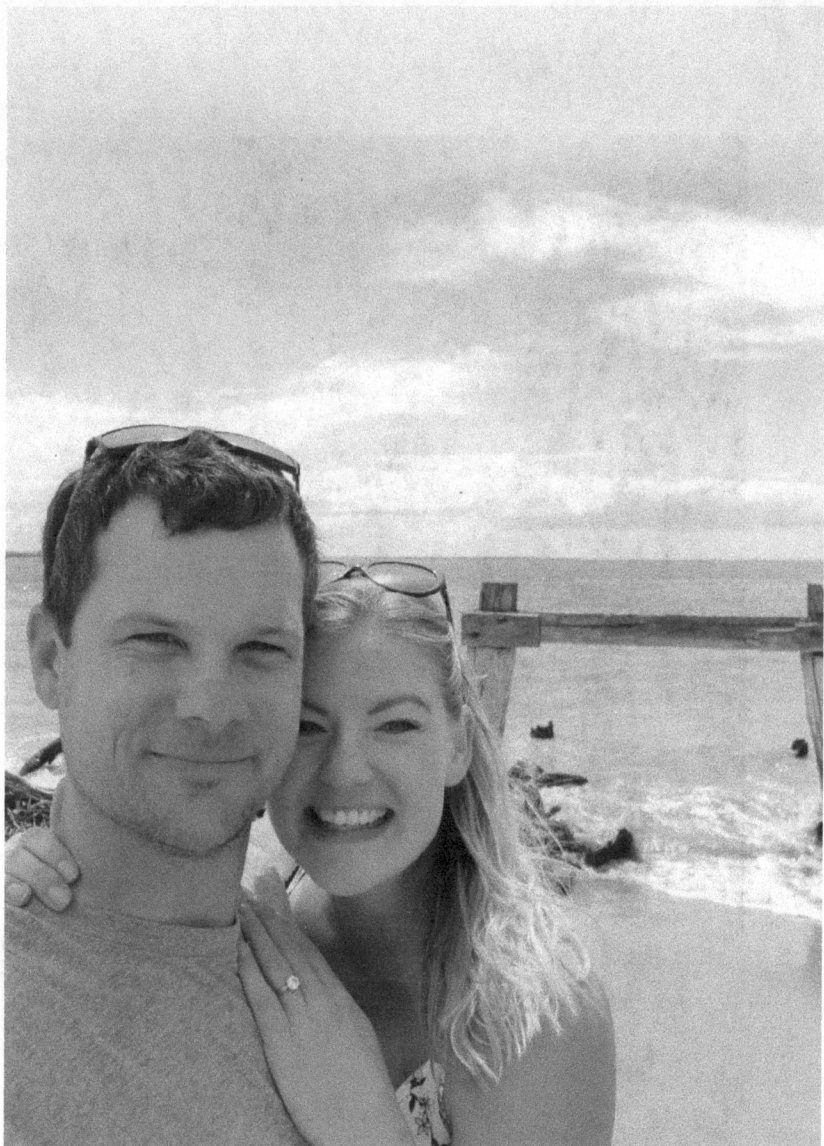

And then this happened... Jem and Mark announce their engagement to friends and family from a beach near Melbourne, five months before their baby's due date.

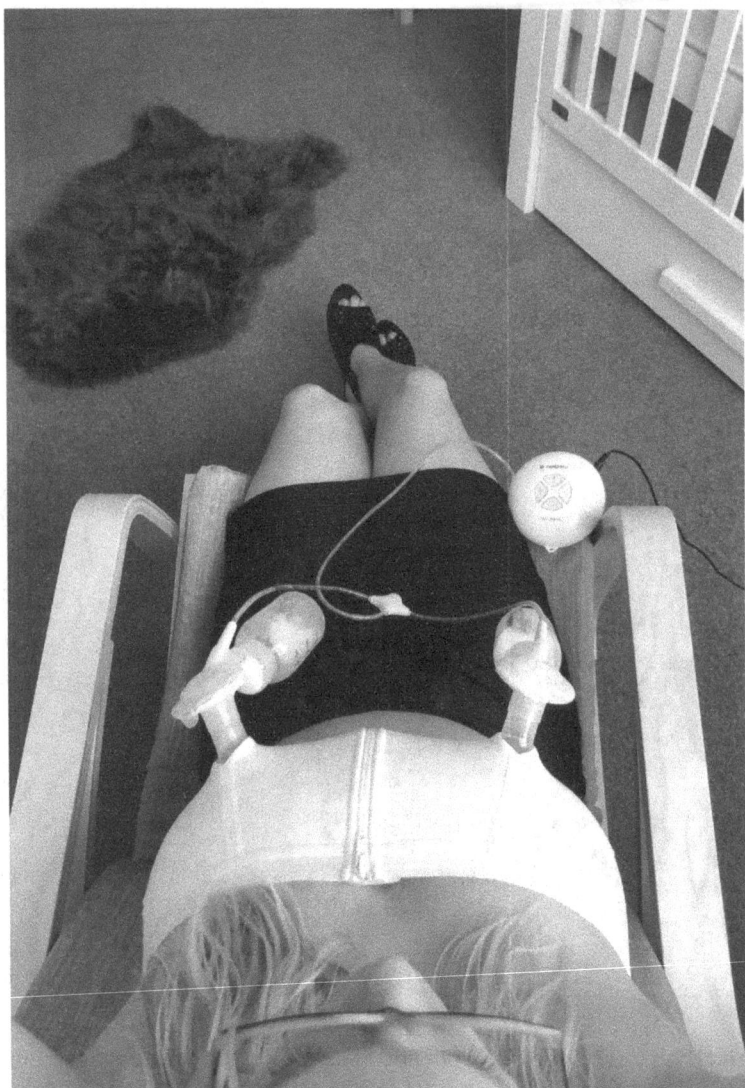

Jem takes time out from court duties to pump in preparation for breastfeeding her daughter. Her midwife recommended she sit in a chair in the future nursery so she could visualise her newborn baby.

# CHAPTER 10

# the birth of Grace

Maddy felt the first twinges of labour at 4am on Thursday, February 28. She was five days past her due date, a pattern with her previous births. Knowing her sister was on tenterhooks, she texted her immediately. When she heard the phone ping, Jem sat up in bed and scanned her sister's words. "Shall we come out now?" she asked. Maddy smiled. If her previous three births were anything to go by, Jem would have plenty of time to get a few more hours of sleep. "No rush," she texted back. But sleep was out of the question for Jem. She got out of bed and expressed more milk, excited knowing her baby would soon be at her breast.

The sisters had discussed their birth plan down to the finest detail: who would be there, when would the midwife be phoned, what would happen immediately after the birth; who would catch the baby, and who would cut and tie the umbilical cord. They were in total agreement about a homebirth. Maddy had birthed her two sons at home, following the trauma of Amelia's birth in Australia. She knew she would be better supported and more relaxed in her own environment with a midwife she trusted, and close family around. She also knew how she laboured: short, mild contractions, strengthening in intensity and frequency over the first 24 hours and then the hard grind through to transition. Her son Lachie's labour had lasted 36 hours, with active labour the best part of a day. Secretly, she hoped this labour could be shorter and easier because it was not her own child. "Maybe it could happen today," she thought. But she felt ready for whatever would eventuate. The night before, Joe and the kids had slept in a tent in the garden to give her a good night's sleep.

Jem and Mark arrived at the house at Horotiu mid-morning. The birthing pool was set up in the lounge. Jem took the older kids to school and she and Maddy went for a walk along the Waikato River path. It was a warm, late summer day, and the sisters enjoyed talking about their excitement leading up to the birth. Rose arrived and the three had coffee. Rose watched her daughters with pride. It had been a long journey filled with sadness and joy to get to this stage. She was excited that the day had come, but also concerned about how the labour would progress. She had privately hoped Maddy might choose a birthing centre rather than home in case there were complications. "I knew how hard her labours were. I had been at Lachie and Harry's births. This was her fourth baby and they live out of town. I was anxious for her wellbeing." But Maddy was adamant that home was best so Rose kept her concerns hidden.

By evening, the contractions were 10 minutes apart and getting stronger, but Maddy knew it was still too early to call Karene. From her midwifery training, she knew a midwife needed to have her sleep before the hard work began. There was already a small group in the house, including Joe, Mark and Rose and Amanda, a close friend and photographer there to capture the birth. "None of these people made me feel uncomfortable," Maddy says, "but they did ask me often how I was doing and whether the contractions were getting closer." At one stage she went to the bedroom to try to get some sleep. Mark and Jem made up a bed for the night and Rose took the boys back to her house, where they would stay until after the birth. Amelia stayed to support her mum, just as Jem and Maddy had done for the births of their brothers.

By 9am on Friday, March 1, the contractions were 2-3 minutes apart. Maddy was doing well, but there were small niggles of worry playing on her mind. As the cervix nears dilation, a small part, known as an anterior lip, can get caught between the cervix and the baby's head. This had happened with her older son Lachie's birth, prolonging labour by several hours. Maddy knew she might still have a long stretch of labouring ahead and she was already tired. While her support team was helping her through the contractions, she knew she needed her confident and reassuring midwife by her side. At 9.30am, Jem phoned Karene.

Karene is an experienced midwife, and a strong proponent of home birth. She has lost count of the number of births she has attended. "Possibly over a thousand." When she began her training in 1986 midwives had to work with GPs, but in 1990, the laws were changed and midwifery became autonomous. For Karene – one of seven children - birth had always been a familiar, joyous, and natural event. She had been at the birth of her twin sister's first baby and, with the help of a midwife, caught her as she birthed. Her own first child, a daughter, was born in her lounge with two midwives and her husband present. "A friend who was a GP was also there, but he sat at the kitchen table and watched." When her daughter was nine months old, she oversaw her first home birth, while her twin sister helped out with childcare. She believes for well women home birth without medical intervention is always best. "She [the woman] is in her own environment, with her partner and possibly family. The midwife is a visitor in her space, not the other way around." There are physiological benefits, too. Oxytocin ("known as 'the hormone of love', because it makes us feel good"), helps with uterus contractions and efficient labours and also in the birthing of the placenta. She says, "Women giving birth at home are less likely to be fearful and produce adrenalin, which isn't conducive to smooth labours. When the birth is over, they can climb into their own bed with their own baby."

Her relationship with Maddy had begun with the birth of Lachie. Maddy was studying midwifery during her pregnancy and was determined her second birth would be different to her daughter's birth by caesarean section in hospital in Australia. She wanted a VBAC (vaginal birth after caesarean), but at Amelia's birth she had been told she had CPD (cephalopelvic disproportion) in which the baby's head was considered too big to fit through her pelvis. She had also been told there were risks that her uterus could rupture. Karene was supportive of her choice and confident she would be able to give birth naturally. "Maddy knew what had happened with Amelia wasn't right. She was determined to try to do things differently. I was very happy to support her choice." Leading up to the birth, a firm trust developed between the two women. When Lachie – nearly half a kilogram heavier than Amelia at birth – was naturally birthed in his parents' lounge after 36 hours' labour, Karene was there to catch him. She was also present for Harry's birth two and a half years later.

Karene was looking forward to being at Maddy's fourth birth. But this was her first surrogate birth, so there were different dynamics in the mix. She had to ensure everyone was comfortable with every decision that had to be made. They also had to know that, for her, Maddy's wellbeing and needs were the highest priority even though the child was not biologically hers. Karene had met Jem previously at Lachie and Harry's births, and knew about her experience with cancer. She also knew Jem shared a similar philosophy with Maddy about home birth. But she didn't know Mark's views. "For babies to be born well, they must be in the place where a woman wants to give birth. Even though this was Jem and Mark's baby, to do well physiologically, as far as Maddy's body was concerned, Maddy needed to be in an environment that worked for her." When Maddy was 33 weeks' pregnant, Karene met Mark to go over the birth process. "I kept sharing that it was normal and safe." Mark was convinced by her assurance and knowing from Jem that this was the way Maddy birthed best.

Karene also met Maddy on her own so she could talk about any mental or emotional issues she might have felt uncomfortable talking about in front of Jem. And she spoke to Jem about the same things. "It felt very safe because of the relationship Jem and Maddy have. They were so open with each other; everything had been discussed." One of the issues the couple had to consider was the moment immediately after the birth. Karene knew Jem would be desperate to hold the baby she had waited for so long. But she also knew the baby should have skin-to-skin contact with the birthing mother to trigger the birth of the placenta and prevent blood loss. Jem didn't hesitate. She knew Maddy's health was a higher priority than her need to hold her baby. She and Mark also agreed Maddy would give the baby her first feed of the rich and highly nutritious colostrum brimming with components that build immunity. When she had drunk her fill, Jem would feed her for the first time. Mark would tie and cut the umbilical cord, using a muka (flax fibres known for their antibacterial properties, which help with healing).

When Karene arrived at the house at 10.25 on March 1, Maddy's contractions were strong, but irregular. Karene was surprised by the number of people at the house. Apart from Maddy, Joe, Jem and Mark, there were Rose, Amelia and Amanda, who was discreetly snapping pictures. A student midwife was due to arrive in a few hours, plus the back-up midwife, which would bring the number to 10. She knew, for many women, being "watched" wasn't conducive to progressing labour. Maddy wasn't concerned by the numbers, but she was definitely over the birth. "I'm confident labouring, but I was totally exhausted and frustrated that we weren't there yet," she says. Jem, Amelia, and Rose took turns rubbing her back in the birthing pool; Joe spoke quietly to his wife, telling her what a great job she was doing. At one stage the couple disappeared into the bedroom to have some quiet time.

At Maddy's request, Karene gave her a herbal tincture to try to regulate the contractions. She also used a "manteada" technique practised in Mexico in which a "rebozo" or scarf or shawl is draped over the woman's hips, which are then gently jiggled from side to side to try to progress the labour. Maddy shifted from position to position, sometimes lying across a Swiss ball, trying to get some relief. At 11am Karene did a vaginal exam. Maddy was just 5-6cm dilated. It was going to be a long afternoon. "Just take me to hospital," said Maddy, a standard request in her other pregnancies very close to the end of labour. When the same thing had happened at Harry's birth, Karene had told her the baby would be born on the side of the road. She advised

Maddy to try to sleep and left for a break, asking Jem to call her when Maddy woke. Joe stroked his wife's back while she slept.

Two hours later, Maddy woke to strong and regular contractions lasting 60 seconds and two to three minutes apart. Jem phoned Karene, who returned immediately. Amelia held her mother's hand. She knew this baby wasn't going to be staying with them, but she also wanted to help. At 3.20 Maddy asked Karene to break her waters. Mark and Jem watched in awe, finding it hard to watch Maddy in such discomfort. "I couldn't believe she was doing this for us," says Jem.

At 4pm, Maddy complained of feeling sick, usually a sign of transition. Karene told her to breathe for 15 minutes. Three-quarters of an hour later Maddy cried, "She's coming." A tiny head crowned and then then a body shot out into Jem's arms to be lifted on to Maddy's tummy. Grace Madeleine Sherson looked straight into her parents' faces. Mark touched her head. When it came time to cut the cord, he tied the beautiful flax muka with gentle hands, his first "dad job" for his daughter. He marvelled at the wonder of witnessing a birth and at the strength of the woman who had carried their child.

Maddy looked down at the baby now feeding hungrily from her breast. She had wondered during the pregnancy what this moment would feel like. Surrogacy is a delicate arrangement with high stakes and high emotions. Would she be emotionally attached to the baby she had birthed? Would she be reluctant to relinquish her? Jem and Mark were prepared to stay longer at the house if that is what she wanted. She looked at Grace's tiny blonde head. Her own newborn babies had had shocks of dark hair. She said, "You are so not my baby", adding "She was the spitting image of Mark." Later, she would say there wasn't a single second of attachment. "It just wasn't an issue. My brain and body never got confused. From the time of the transplant, I always thought of Grace as my niece, and that didn't change when she was born. I wish I'd known that from the start." She knows there is curiosity and some concern among the general public about the emotional transfer of a surrogate baby to the parents and that some surrogates worry they will find it hard. The questions she was most asked when she was pregnant were, "How could you give your baby up? How will you cope? Won't it be hard?" She and Jem had talked about those concerns. But none eventuated. "I always knew I was babysitting. The love I have for my own babies is entirely different. I didn't experience a single minute of loss when Grace was given to Jem and Mark." She hopes her experience will put other potential surrogates' minds at rest.

For Jem, seeing her baby suckling at her sister's breast was a magical experience. "It was just so overwhelming. I never thought of snatching Grace out of Maddy's arms. It felt like it was still part of the birth. I enjoyed seeing her feeding Grace. It wasn't time to give her to me until it was time to give her to me." Grace fed from Maddy for about 45 minutes and Jem says that positive experience set her up to succeed. "She was so relaxed." After she was weighed (she was 4.25kg, bigger than Maddy's own three babies at birth), Jem took her newborn daughter in her arms and felt her latch on to her own breast. "I couldn't believe I was feeding her." Tears well up. "It makes me so emotional. It's amazing that your body can do that. It made that attachment so raw and so real. I looked down at my huge boobs and there was this little head nestling there. She was just feeding. It was incredible. It was the highlight of the birth." For the new parents, the birth was the beginning of a new chapter. When Jem was ill, they had focused their thoughts on a future of happiness beyond the disease. It was what sustained Jem on the nights she wept in Mark's arms about not being able to carry her own child. Grace was proof her hopes had come true. She says the gratitude they have for Maddy knows no bounds. "She helped create our family."

Maddy was also euphoric. She was pleased and relieved the labour had gone to plan and loved watching her sister bond with her baby. But she was utterly exhausted and looked forward to collapsing in her own bed without being woken for feeds. That night she would sleep for 14 hours...

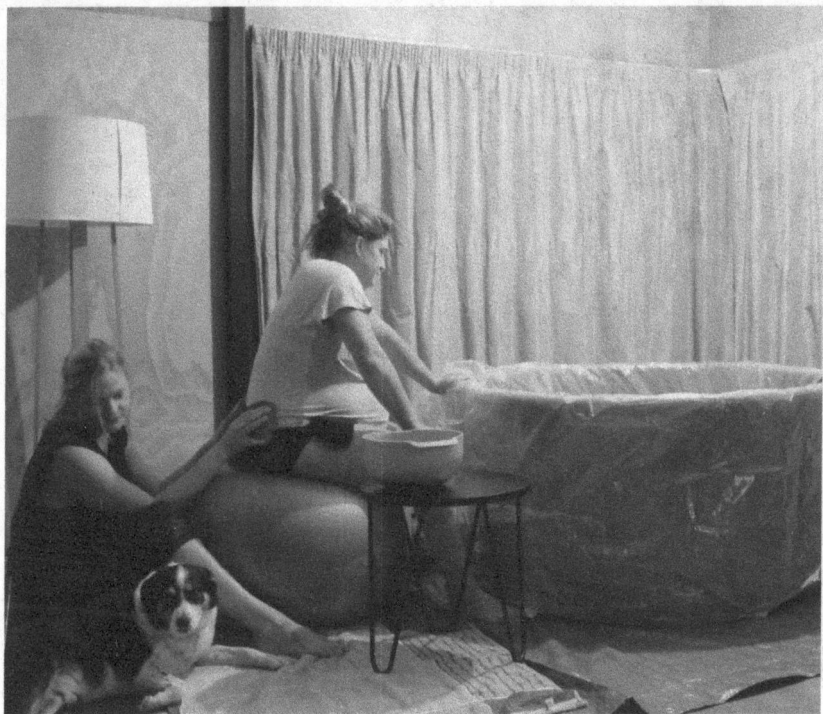

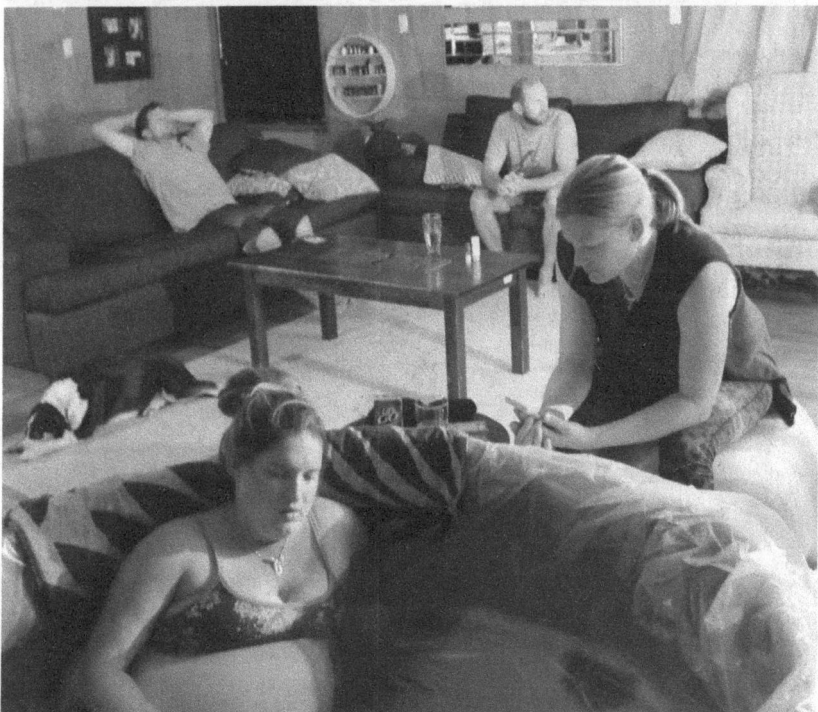

A birthing bath is set up in Maddy and Joe's living room.

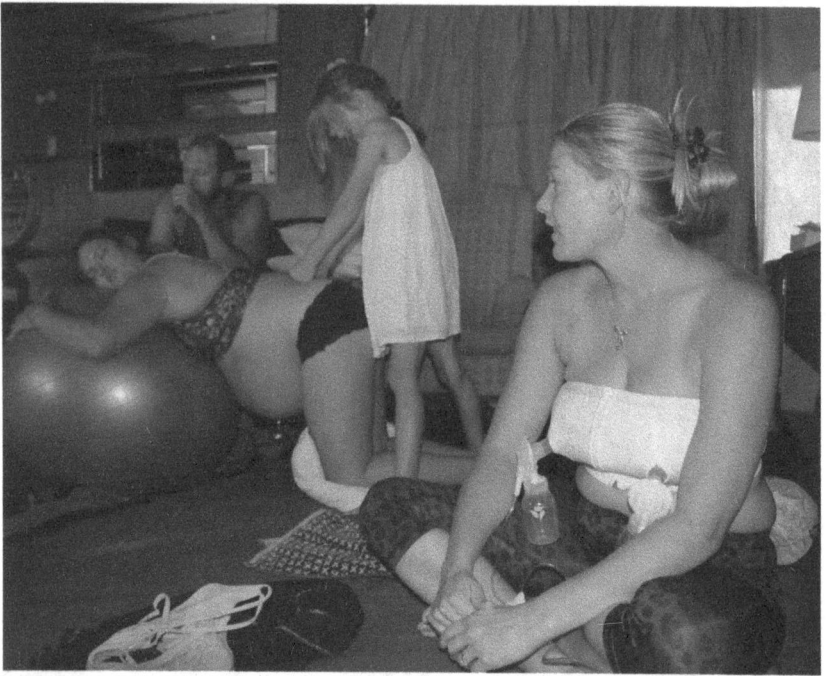

Jem continues to pump as Amelia massages her mother's back.

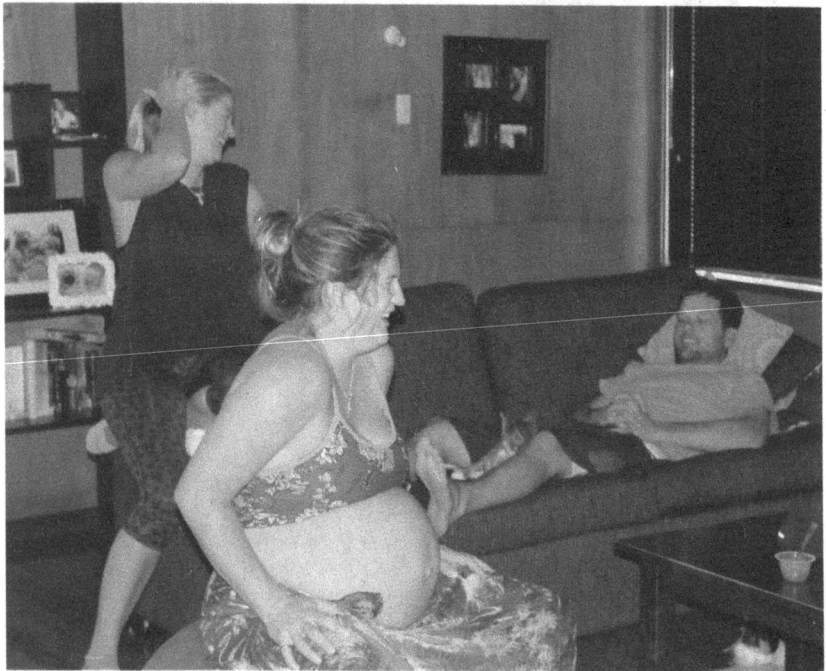

There are moments of humour, but Maddy is getting tired as the labour progresses.

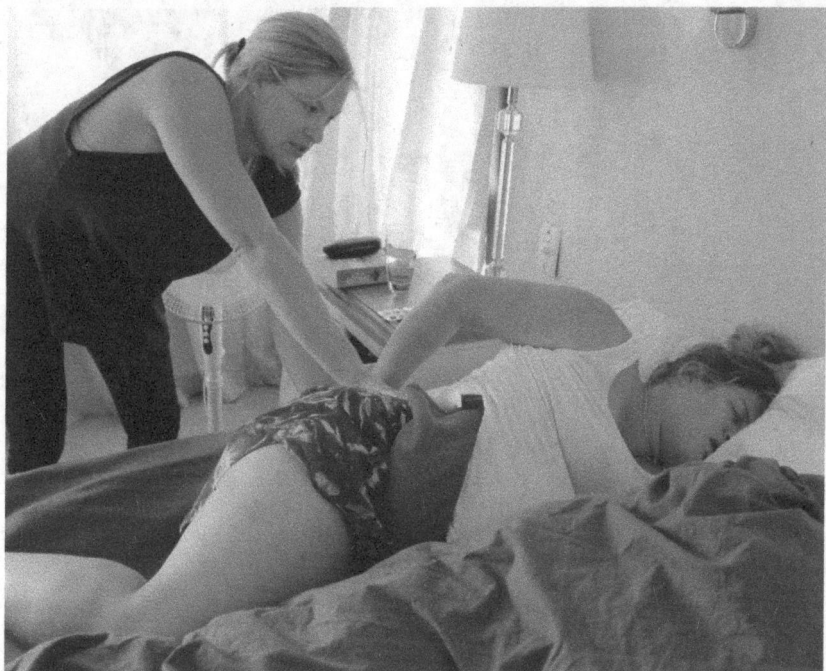

Jem massages her sister's back.

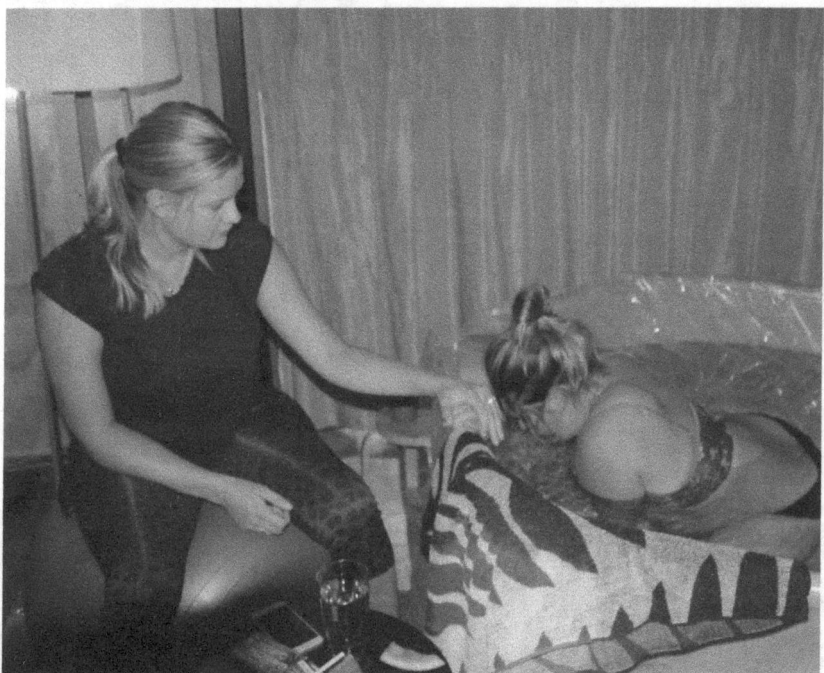

Jem holds Maddy's hand in the pool as the labour intensifies.

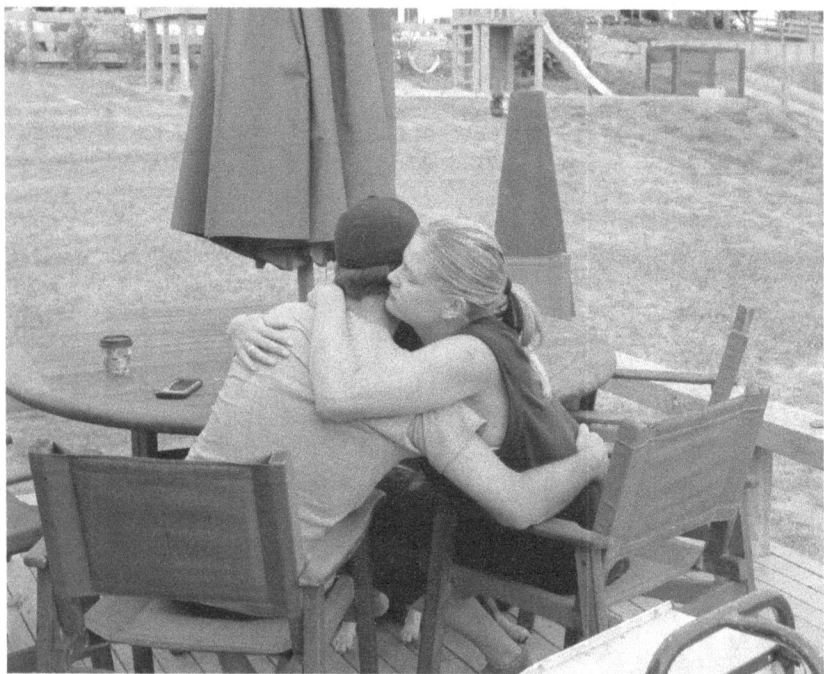

Mark and Jem take some time for a quiet moment.

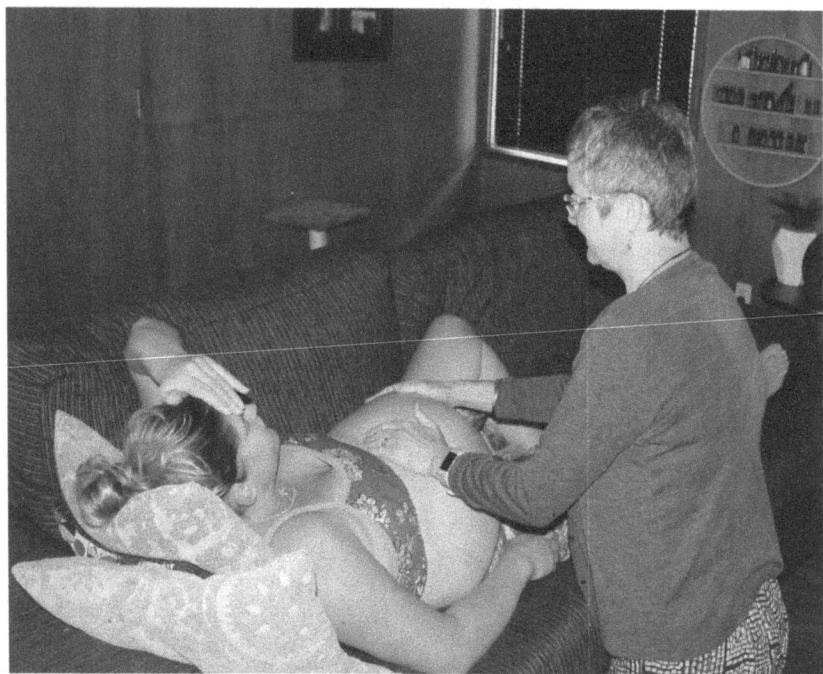

Midwife Karene checks the baby's progress.

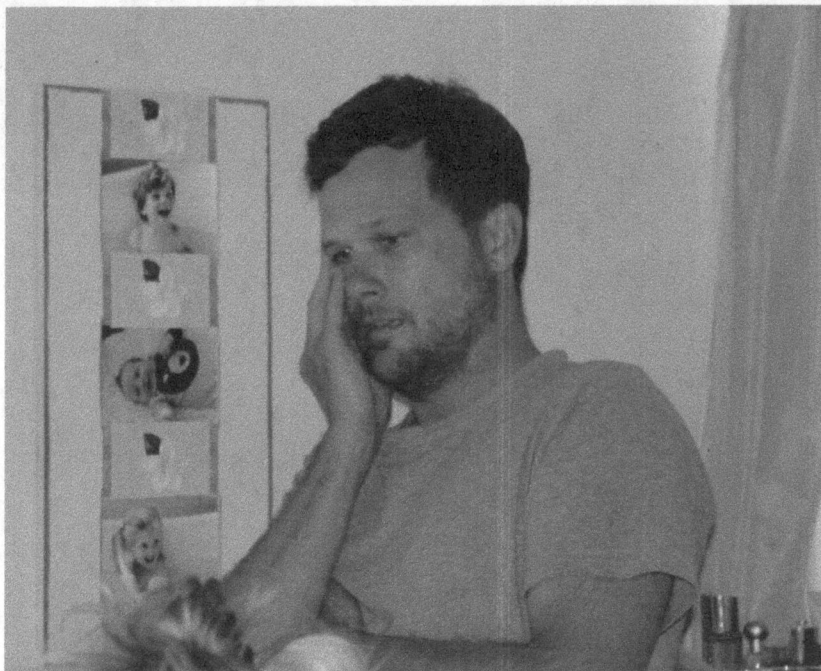

Mark watches in awe as his daughter is born.

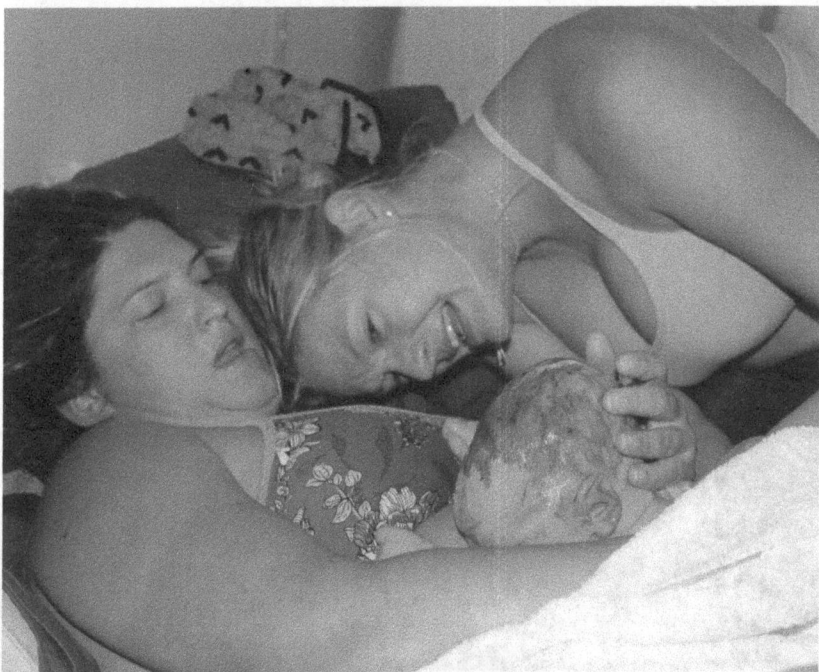

Jem sees her daughter for the first time.

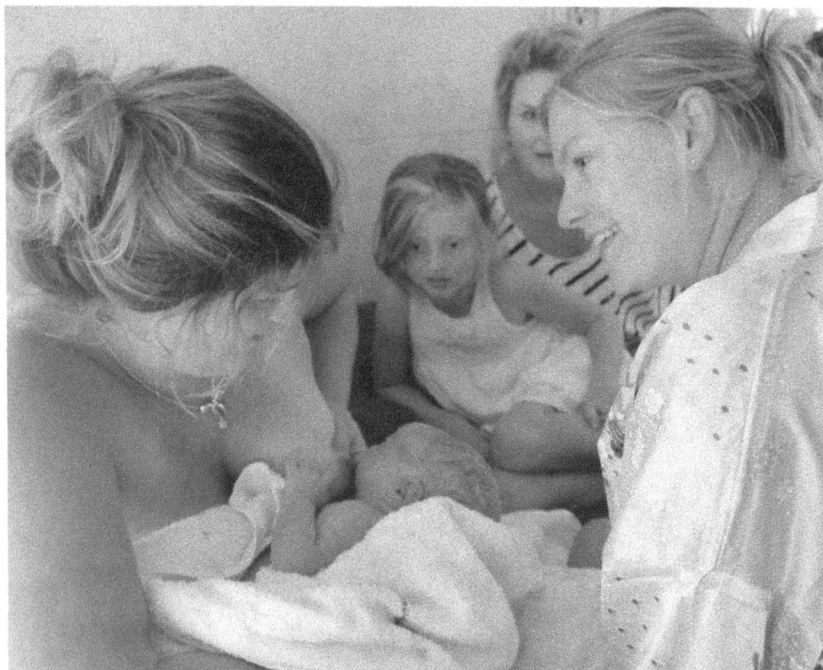

Maddy gives Grace her first feed, watched by Jem, Amelia, and Rose.

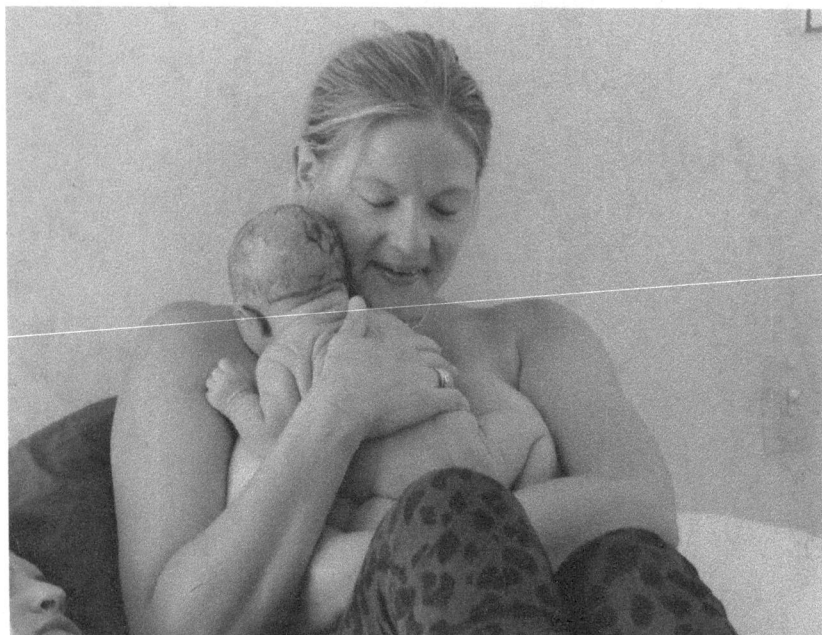

Jem gets first mummy cuddles.

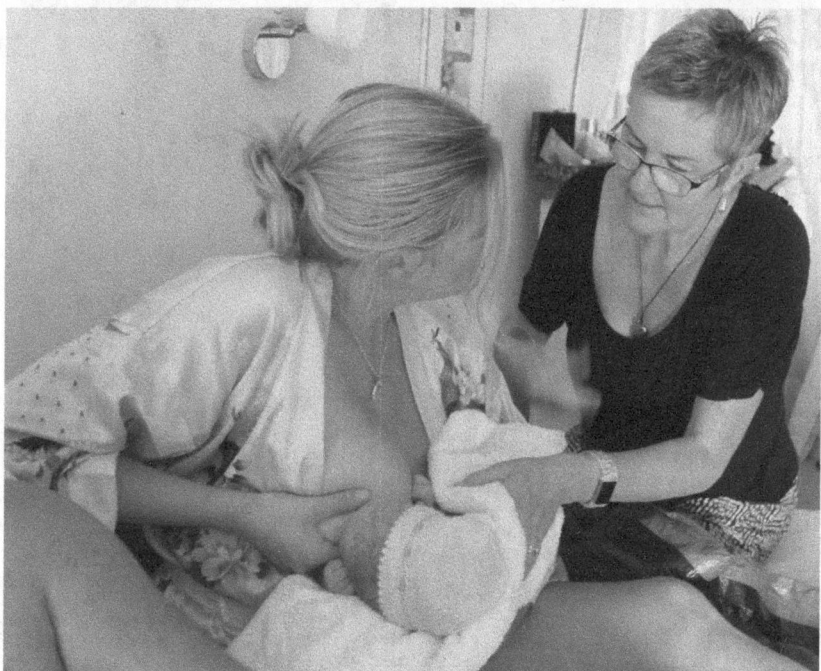

"I couldn't believe I was feeding her." Karene helps Jem get Grace to latch on.

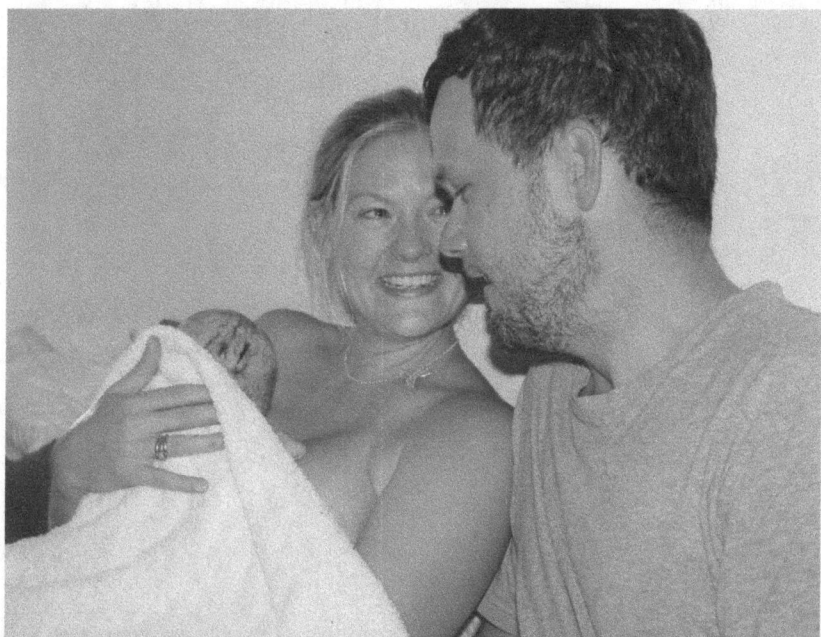

Mark and Jem enjoy their first moments as parents of Grace.

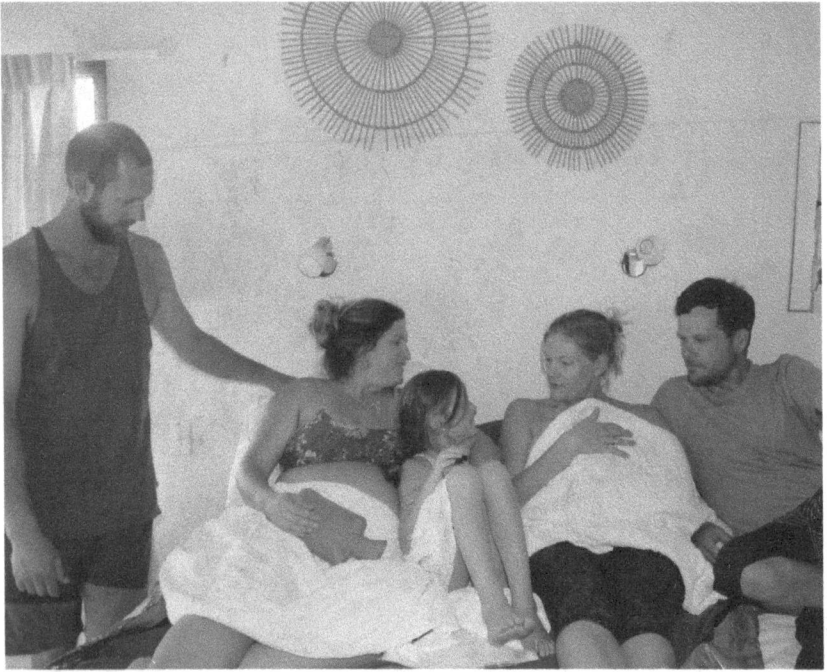

We are family. Joe, Maddy, Amelia, Jem, Mark, and Grace.

# CHAPTER 11

# Sleepless nights and a scare

While Maddy was sleeping deeply, Mark and Jem were adjusting to their first night as new parents. They had booked in for two nights at the Waterford Birthing Centre, so Jem could have support to establish feeding. They were still on a post-birth high as the night drew in. But, as most parents will attest, parenting has its ups and downs. For three nights, Grace Madeline Sherson, a picture perfect baby who they had craved for more than two years, yelled her head off through the night. Jem was distraught and Mark was concerned. But Maddy was sanguine. "Just normal baby stuff," she texted her sister. To help Jem have a break, she fed Grace and rocked her to sleep, assuring her sister that every first-time parent finds the going tough. She also offered to continue to pump milk for the next 12 weeks to bolster Jem's supply.

Breastfeeding a newborn takes patience and confidence. Jem had plenty of patience but worried that Grace wasn't getting enough milk. For the first few days, she needed only around 50mls a feed, but when her demand picked up, she overtook Jem's supply. To prevent her milk supply slipping, Jem pumped between feeds. "It felt like my boobs had been taken over and I was just a production line." Nights and days merged into each other as mother and baby adjusted to changing routines. Mark moved into the spare room and Jem co-slept with Grace so she could feed her on demand when she was hungry or distressed. She learned to differentiate her cries. Friends appeared with gifts and words of love and encouragement – and advice. Mark reassured her she was doing a fantastic job. She says, "I'd look at this small bundle that we had wanted so much and feel so guilty that I was feeling stressed." Like most parents all she craved was sleep.

Karene became her confidante and biggest fan. She talked to her for hours, reassuring her that she was doing well. Jem kept a feeding journal, showing how much milk she was giving Grace, whether it was frozen or directly from the breast, and how long she fed on each side: columns and columns of notations that Karene could check. She used all the devices to encourage Grace to continue to suckle from the breast: finger feeding (essentially a glorified straw that encourages the baby to suckle expressed milk at the breast), lactate tubes taped to her breasts and even sippy cups. Each day she would review her progress. "I wanted to get to six months at least." Her support team assured her she could quit at any time, but she grew more determined to persist. At six months, she looked at her healthy, but still hungry baby and introduced some supplementary feeding from the bottle. Mum and baby thrived.

Almost every new mother will have a similar story about the first year of their child's life. There are the highlights – less waking during the night; the joy of seeing a baby roll over or laugh – the lowlights of teething and changes to sleeping habits just when you think you have it sussed. Jem and Mark were no different. Over the first months of Grace's life, they learned to work as a team in parenthood, supporting each other if they felt low, and celebrating the milestones of parenthood. When Grace was just over six months, they were looking forward to their first real holiday as a family. A close friend was getting married in the Cook Islands. A few weeks before the wedding, a measles epidemic spread through New Zealand, causing parents of new-borns to worry they would come in contact with unvaccinated children. People with children were warned not to gather in airports. Jem and Mark consulted their GP. Should they cancel their travel plans? Could Grace be vaccinated? Most children don't have their measles inoculation until they are one. The advice was to have it done early if you intend travelling.

Grace was vaccinated and three days later came out in a rash that covered her body. Her temperature rocketed and she was clearly unwell. Jem was beside herself, worried that this precious baby they had fought so hard to bring into the world might have a serious disease. She rang the GP who arranged to check the baby in the carpark beside the clinic to avoid any contamination. As he approached in full protective gear, Jem looked at Grace stripped down to her nappy in the back of the car. "She looked so vulnerable." The doctor gently pushed his thumb into the rash. "Not measles," he said. "Probably a reaction to the vaccination." He recommended Pamol and lots of liquids. Three days later, the family boarded a plane to the Cook Islands for a welcome break in the sun.

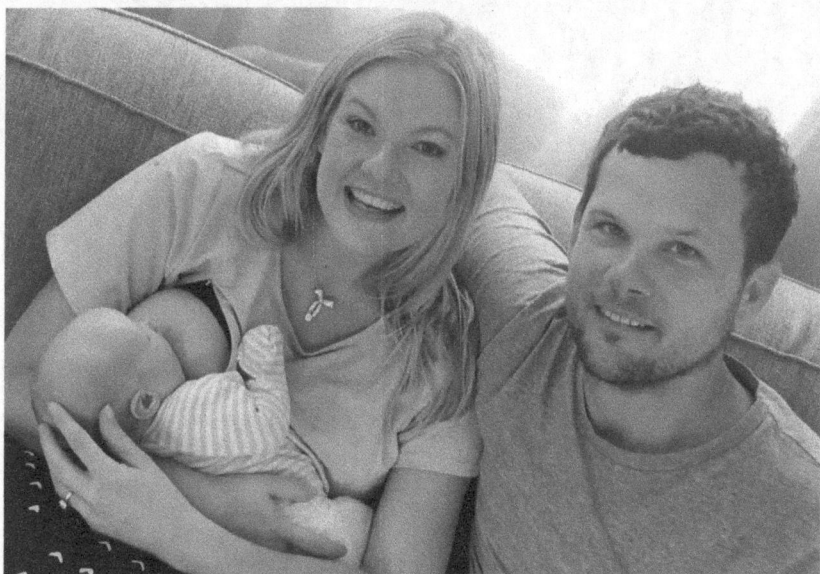
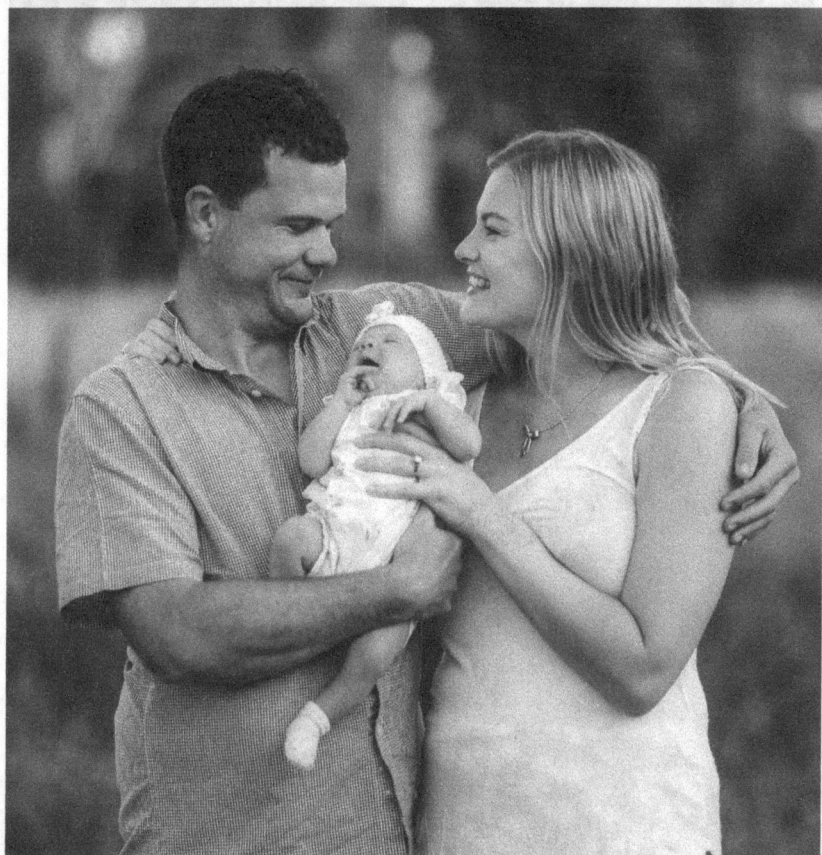

And baby makes three. Back home with Grace.

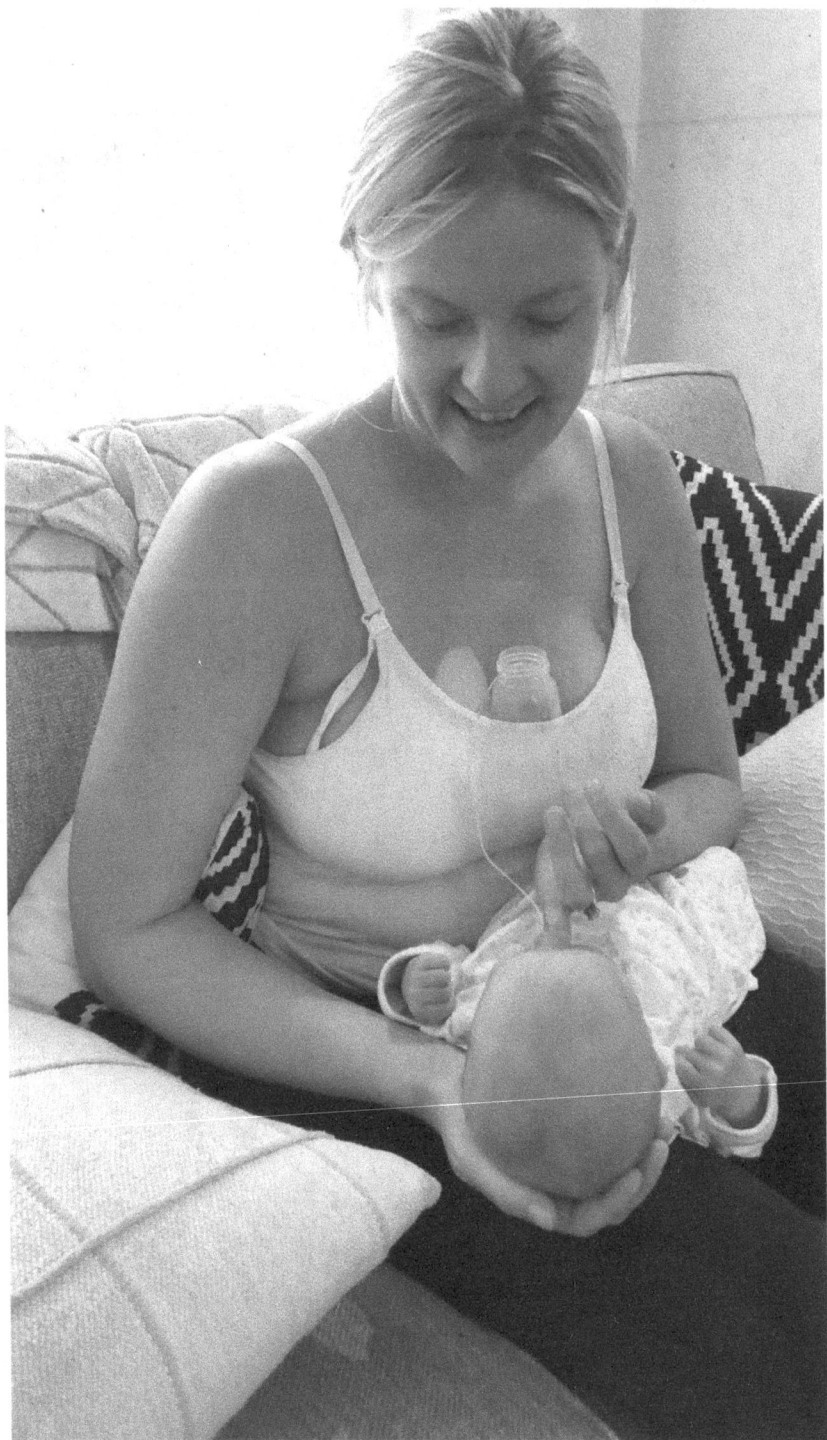

Finger feeding to encourage suckling.

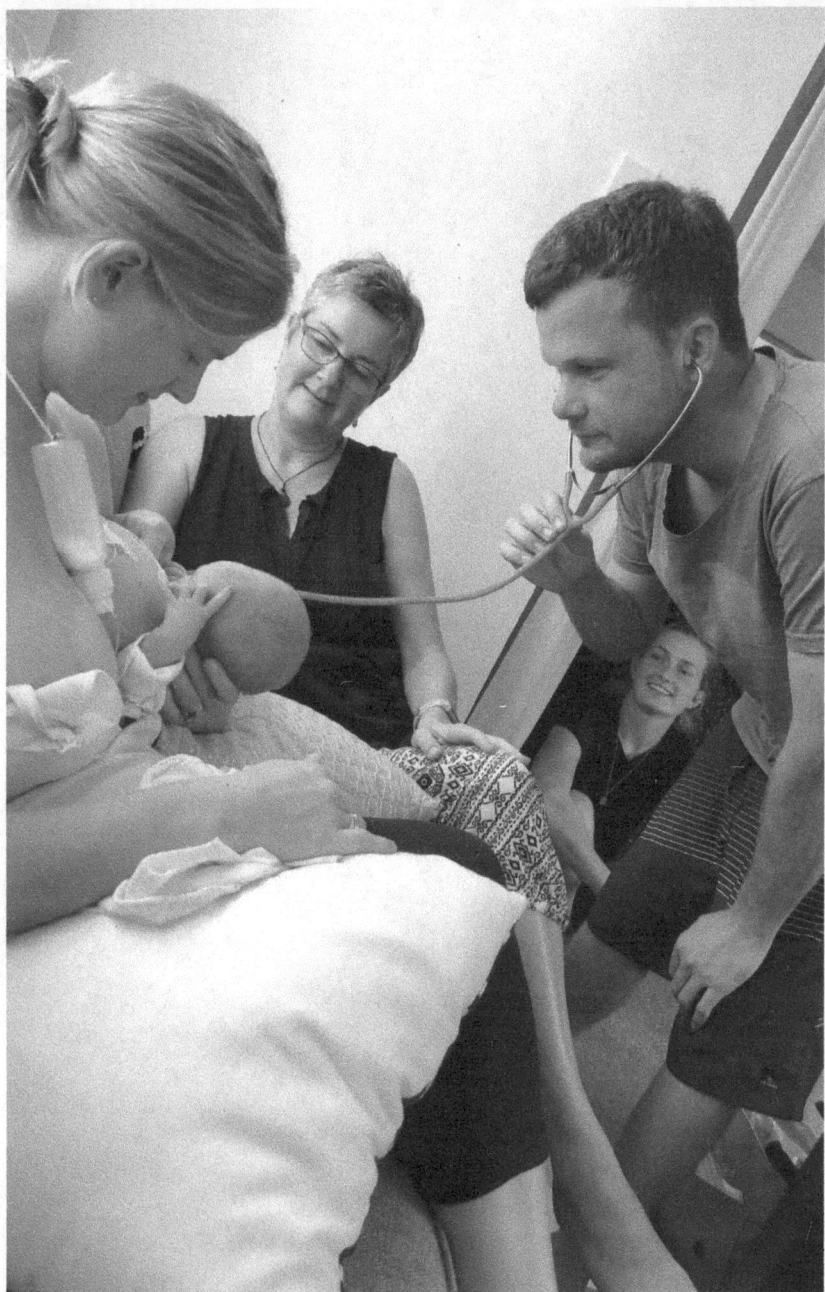

Yes, I can breastfeed. Karene supports Jem in ways to feed Grace, watched by Mark and a trainee midwife.

# CHAPTER 12

# Men are not bit players

## Joe's story

Joe Turner is a man of few words. The 35-year-old steel fabricator describes himself as an ordinary guy; reserved unless he has something to say. He works hard, dotes on his three kids, enjoys the occasional weekend hunting or fishing with mates, or sharing a beer around the barbecue of his rural home, overlooking lush farmland north of Hamilton. Like many men he doesn't talk a lot about his feelings.

But, when his wife Maddy, first raised the subject of being a surrogate for her sister and her partner, he didn't miss a beat. "It didn't surprise me Maddy made the offer. She and Jem are incredibly close, and Jem is very special to all of us. I just thought, 'That makes sense'. And that was it." Nearly two years after the initial offer was made, his views haven't changed.

"I am so proud of Maddy, that she was willing to do it. It's an amazing thing, a generous gift. I never doubted her and I never doubted it was the right thing to do."

But Joe is not typical of all men whose wives want to be a surrogate. For many, the thought of their wife carrying another couple's baby is abhorrent. With no biological ties to the children their wives are carrying, they worry about how they will cope with a pregnancy they had nothing to do with. There are other things to consider: abstinence from sex during the implantation; a woman's hormonal fluctuations during a pregnancy that does not result in their own child; the risks to their wives during the pregnancy plus any impact of relinquishing the child at birth. There may also be financial stresses. In New Zealand, surrogates aren't paid, and any financial rewards offered by the intended parents are limited to the necessities of pregnancy and birth. Surrogates often have to delay a return to work or take time off work during the pregnancy, meaning their earning capacity is put on hold.

While women's surrogacy stories are commonly shared, husbands' views are often overlooked, or they are included as bit players. But what is known is that not all men react positively to their wives' proposal. Some refuse point plank to agree, leading to stress and occasionally divorce if they can't resolve their differences.

Joe wasn't fazed. "I don't tend to worry about things in advance." But he does think having a solid relationship and talking through any issues is key to success. The couple had already decided Maddy would not return to work while she was breastfeeding their youngest child, Harry. It made sense for her to try to get pregnant with Jem and Mark's baby immediately after Harry weaned. She had been healthy during previous pregnancies and given birth without problems. Joe knew she would be physically tired with three young children. He knew that he would be working away from home at times during her pregnancy, which could put added strain on Maddy. But he also knew she was resilient. The overwhelming consideration was that this was something life-changing they could do for Jem. Joe has huge affection for his sister-in-law and they have been close friends since school days, when he and Maddy started dating. He is also committed to family life and realised the pleasure children could bring to a relationship. He wanted Jem to have that with Mark. It helped greatly to have a friendship with Mark, whom he liked and believed would be a good dad.

"When Maddy put it to me formally, of course I said 'yes'."

While the surrogacy was the focus of a lot of conversations between the two couples in the lead-up to the first embryo transplant, the men never discussed it privately. "Mark's like me, he doesn't share his feelings with people he doesn't know well." But during counselling with Fertility Associates, both men were asked to consider their responses to a range of scenarios to test their reactions. When Joe was asked what he would do if anything happened to Jem and Mark during the pregnancy, he answered immediately, "Well, we'd keep it (the baby) wouldn't we?"

The first stress came when Maddy suffered a miscarriage after the first embryo implant. She was upset, thinking she had let Jem down. As they approached the second implant, Joe tried not to focus on the possibility of another disappointment. But, like Maddy, he was ecstatic when the pregnancy was confirmed. Over the next nine months, there were other stresses. He was working in Hokitika on and off during winter. Maddy would ring him to vent when she was tired or the children were playing up. At one stage, he suggested they sit down with Jem and Mark to discuss how she could be better supported. "They (Jem and Mark) came up with some practical ideas to support her with the kids. It all changed then."

There were some light-hearted moments, too. When men who didn't know the couple congratulated Joe on Maddy being pregnant, he would comment, "Yeah, but it's not mine." Once they had recovered from their shock, he would explain about the surrogacy arrangement. "They were always interested."

As the birth neared, he prepared himself to support Maddy, whom he knew had long and powerful labours. He had marvelled at her strength during the births of their own children, but he knew how tired she would be. There were also more people involved. He wondered how she would cope. "I took my cues from her. If she had asked me to clear the room, I would have done so, but she was okay with it."

While it was hard to watch her experiencing painful contractions, he reminded himself this was "a chosen struggle", not like the pain of an illness. He stroked her back and told her continuously how well she was doing. When Grace was born, he felt a tremendous burst of pride for what they had accomplished. And relief. "I had always thought of the baby as my niece, and it didn't change when she was born. I was just so pleased that we had reached our goal."

## Mark's story

Mark Sherson is also a man of few words. But the 39-year-old landscaper doesn't hold back when it comes to describing his feelings about the gift Maddy and Joe offered when they suggested Maddy could carry their child. When the offer was made, he and Jem had weathered the toughest period of their relationship. He had seen Jem frightened by her cancer prognosis and despairing of her inability to carry their child. He had watched her rage at the unfairness of it all. "We hadn't had time to talk much about the future when she became ill," he says. "But I knew she was special. Her sadness after the diagnosis and the operation was hard to watch. I had experienced nothing at that level." For months, he saw her vent privately when they were alone, while trying to carry on her life outside. He held her when she cried and stroked her hair. He told her over and over her life was worth more than any child they could have had together. "I already had a son, so I didn't perhaps feel it so intensely, but I wanted it to happen for her. I knew she would be a wonderful mother and I knew how much family meant to her."

He knew little about surrogacy at the start. But as time progressed he realised what a massive deal it was for Maddy to step forward. "Initially, I thought of it as a sisterly thing, the arrangement between the two women." But as he got more involved and underwent counselling with Fertility Associates, he appreciated the magnitude of his sister and brother-in-law's commitment to him and Jem having their own child.

When the first implant resulted in a miscarriage, he again held Jem as she mourned the loss. "I knew it was bad news, but I also knew the success rates and I guess I had prepared myself for what happened." But, like Jem, he was concerned there was only one more viable embryo. "We talked about the implications if the second implant didn't work. Jem had not long finished her cancer treatment and it would be some time before they could harvest more eggs. We weren't even sure whether that would be successful. Plus, the delay would mean Maddy and Joe would have to weigh up whether they could put their lives on hold for another year. They had planned for Maddy to return to work a year after Harry was born, so they were already looking at a financial impact. To push it out further would have been really difficult."

When the second implant – the last of their frozen embryos – resulted in a successful pregnancy, the joy was indescribable.

"For once, we could really focus on the future." But there were still some stresses. When it became apparent Maddy needed more than just gifts and flowers, he and Jem reassessed their contributions. While Jem helped Maddy in practical ways by cooking and transporting the children to school and sports events, Mark helped Joe build a playground for the children. "The practical help made a huge difference to all of us."

Some men involved in surrogate arrangements say they feel distanced from the pregnancy. Whereas with their own wives, they can share the bodily changes and feel the baby's kicks, it might not seem appropriate to do that with another woman. But Mark says Maddy was hugely generous and shared every change with him and Jem. "Jem was still very sad that she wasn't carrying our child. I told her, 'it's not important that you aren't pregnant with our child; the important thing is that we are having a child'."

He says finding out the sex of their child at the 20-week scan also helped him feel closer to his unborn daughter. "I hadn't thought it was so important to know, but Jem was keen. I'm glad we did because it certainly felt like a closer connection. We could buy things for her and talk about her as a real person."

He and Joe had become good friends, since he started dating Jem "He's a good guy; a really good bugger. We are different but we like the same stuff. He's very straight-up, which I appreciate. And he's a good dad; a good family man." He was also grateful that Joe was so relaxed about the surrogacy. "He didn't make like it was a big deal or that he was doing a big thing by letting his wife carry our child."

On the day of the birth, Mark was excited. He had missed the birth of his son Ethan, so it was new to him. The night before Grace was born he and Jem had little sleep. As he watched Maddy labour throughout the next day, he felt an overwhelming sense of gratitude and wonder at her strength. "It was pretty amazing. I was so happy. Yes, I was tearful. It was a huge relief to hold our daughter." It was also strange for them to leave Maddy and Joe. "We were quite prepared to stay for a few days if that was what Maddy wanted or Jem needed help with breastfeeding. But it was all okay."

As he tucked his newborn daughter into her car seat, the full emotion of what they had been through struck him. He and Jem were to be married. They were a family. A new stage of their life together had begun.

# CHAPTER 13

# the best day

February 15, 2020 was overcast in Tauranga, but the temperature was still in the mid-20s. There was some relief that the burning sun of the previous days was shielded by cloud cover. The staff at Olive Tree Cottage had been up in the cool of the early morning to ready the venue for the event, draping vines and fairy lights along the tables and over a chandelier of entwined deer antlers. Built in the 1930s, Olive Tree Cottage was originally a three-bedroom kauri home on rural land 15 minutes from the city centre. In the 1990s, it was renovated and adapted as a venue for events. The weathered rich dark floors revealed its age, but new features had been added including a silk-draped marquee with a dance floor, a gazebo and rustic garden arch. The gardens, lawns and mature trees were lush despite the summer drought. In the distance, the 232m lava dome, Mauao, a landmark of the beach resort, Mount Maunganui, was visible through the heat haze.

Lisa Pattillo, grand-daughter of Olive Tree Cottage's original owner, Pat Best, cast an expert eye over the preparations. She had catered for dozens of events at the venue and understood each client's need to put their own stamp on proceedings. The sound system had been checked and rechecked; the vines, picked by family and transported from Hamilton the day before had been placed in ice buckets to preserve them. A basket of peppermint-coloured jandals was placed near the dance floor for guests with tired feet. A sign near the wooden benches where guests would sit read: "Pick a seat on either side, you are loved by both groom and bride." Near the gazebo, was a basket of dried rose petals to be thrown by guests. Lisa knew her team was meticulous in their preparation. But for her, this was not just another wedding. She was related to the bridal party by marriage.

At Maungatapu, in a house overlooking Tauranga harbour, the groom and his brother, the best man, were going through the final checklist fortified by coffee from a nearby BP station. The two groomsmen – the groom's 20-year-old son and a good friend – checked their shoes and trouser lengths. One pair was bunching at the ankles so it was whisked off by a competent sister-in-law and hemmed with tape. Suit jackets were checked for fluff and ties straightened. The week before there had been a minor disagreement over whether the groom should wear a waistcoat and bow tie to set him apart from the groomsmen. There was further debate over whether the groomsmen should wear braces. In the end, the groom conceded the waistcoat and bow tie looked sharp, but the braces were shelved.

At Papamoa, on the ocean beach 30 minutes away, the bride was going through her own checklist with her three attendants – her sister, the maid of honour, and two friends. The six-bedroom modern multi-storey apartment, with views out to the Pacific Ocean, was filled to capacity with family and attendants, some sleeping marae-style on mattresses on the floor. Make-up artists and hairstylists went about their work calmly amid the chaos. A photographer kept out of the traffic. The partner of the bride's mother, a winemaker from Marlborough, played music and kept up some light-hearted banter to ease any tension. The bride was excited, but nervous. When she had woken that morning, her sister had passed on a wedding day gift from the groom: a pink crystal, a symbol of serenity and love. She touched it every now and again to remind her of his love.

At 1pm, a limo arrived to pick up the groom's party, pausing while a second photographer captured the men leaving the house. The brothers sat next to each other, the older one reassuring his sibling, again, that he had the rings in his pocket. The older brother remembered his own wedding day in Queenstown, 10 years before and all the last-minute details that had run through his mind. Then the roles had been reversed and he had been grateful for his brother's support and reassurance.

At the venue, guests had begun to arrive. There would be nearly 100 friends and family, people who had known the couple all their lives, others classmates from Hillcrest High School in Hamilton. Some hadn't seen each other for years. There was a lot to catch up on over a glass of champagne.

Just before 3pm, a people mover arrived carrying the flower girls and pageboys. There were five children strapped into their car seats, driven by the woman who would look after them later that night. Amelia, 8, the oldest flower girl, took her role seriously. She had rehearsed the day before and knew she had to lead the bridal party very slowly down the path, plus oversee the younger members – her brothers Lachie, 6 and Harry, 3, and cousin, Chloe, 4.

The youngest flower girl, and the last to be lifted from the car, was Grace Madeleine Sherson aged nearly one. For her parents' wedding, she wore a pale pink broderie anglaise dress, edged with lace hearts. Her hair, the colour of spun gold, lightened by the summer sun, was covered by a straw hat decorated with flowers. Her shoes, which had been carefully matched to her dress, would later be kicked off so she could bounce up and down on the dance floor.

In the gazebo, standing by the groom's party, celebrant Denise Irvine readied herself for the ceremony. She had conducted dozens of weddings, but this event was all the more meaningful because she had also known Mark since birth. Today would also have been her and her late husband Bill's 50th wedding anniversary. Like most guests, she knew this was a particularly poignant day, marking a couple's celebration of love, but also new life and the strength that comes with facing down adversity. She smiled as the best man patted the pocket with the rings and reached forward to tuck in a section of the groom's shirt that had worked loose.

The flower girls and pageboys came first. The girls wore the same pale pink layered frocks as Grace; the boys wore braces over their white shirts, black shorts, and trendy ankle-high brown boots. They walked slowly and seriously towards the gazebo, sneaking shy glances at the faces lining the path, including grandparents, aunts, uncles, and their parents' friends. Amelia focused hard on the place where they would stand at the end of the path while the ceremony took place. She knew if anyone was fidgety, her job was to remind them to be quiet.

The first senior attendant to appear was the maid of honour Madeleine Turner, Jem's sister, mother of Amelia, Lachie, and Harry and "Aunty Mum" to Grace, followed by her sister-in-law Tracey Turner (mother of flower girl Chloe), and second bridesmaid Janine Van De Pas, whose work in planning this wedding would later be acknowledged.

On her last day as Jemani Alice Alchin-Boller, the bride walked down the path on the arm of her father, Henry, to the sound of *Amazing Grace*, sung by Tigirlily, a Nashville duo of sisters. It was a song that captured the joy and wonder of her daughter's birth. She wore a slim-fitting, strapless lace dress covered with glass sequins, a narrow veil pinned to her blonde hair and a smile that took in the guests, but which was directed at Mark, the man whom she would later describe to guests as her best friend, love of her life and the rock that had kept her steady for the past three years.

Mark watched her as she walked down the path. It was a surreal moment. They had been through so much together and he was overcome by the thought that they would now be husband and wife. "You look beautiful, bub," he said as she stepped up beside him. Denise Irvine smiled at the couple holding hands and reminded the guests to reflect for a moment on what marriage meant. "Marriage is based on love," she said, "but it also offers close friendship; it is an anchor in rough seas." She added, "Jem has said she has never felt the absolute security that she feels with Mark. She says Mark has been her strength through the best and worst times." During their vows, Mark and Jem promised to be lifelong companions, to build dreams together, rejoice in times of happiness and support each other in times of trouble. When they exchanged rings and kissed for the first time as husband and wife, the guests erupted with cheers. But there was one final ceremony to come. To signify the importance of their family, the couple presented Mark's son Ethan with a pounamu toki (adze), signifying strength, control, and determination. For their daughter Grace, they chose a heart-shaped silver locket. Denise Irvine quoted American writer James McBride, who wrote, "Family is like the wind: instinctive, raw, fragile, beautiful, at times angry, but always unstoppable. It is our collective breath. It is the world's greatest force. It is our last miracle." Then she turned to the guests. "Please give our warmest congratulations to our newly married couple, Jem and Mark Sherson."

On the grass below, Amelia took her cue to rally the young attendants as the bridal party began their walk back down the path. The rose petals she had earlier handed to guests caught on the breeze and landed softly on the shoulders of the bride and groom. The newlyweds held hands and raised their arms in sheer joy as they walked back down the path.

Later that evening, there was more laughter as speakers shared anecdotes about the couple as children and young adults. There was a story about Jem, as a teenager, cutting Maddy's waist-length hair to a short, uneven bob above her ears; the groom's brother quoted Section 10B of the Crimes Act, 1961, which he said set a 10-year limitation period in respect to any legal action the groom might want to take "for multiple threats of grievous bodily harm, and tying him to the staircase when we were young." But there were also references to the toughest time in the couple's relationship when Jem was diagnosed with cancer a few months into their relationship. Maddy talked about her sister's fortitude and determination to push through the dark times and refusal to give up on her dreams. She described her sister as her idol and protector: "the one who has always been there for me." She also paid tribute to Mark as he rode the rollercoaster of Jem's emotions, during the year following her treatment. "I once had to literally sit on Jem's phone to stop her venting to Mark. She was trying to push him away to test his commitment. I thought he will surely run for the hills. But he didn't. It was then I knew he was a keeper."

Sam also acknowledged his brother's quiet strength and qualities as a father and now husband. He also revealed a secret not known by many outside Jem's family, that she had had a secret crush on Mark when they were at school. Mark, in his speech admitted later, "If someone had told me at school that I would one day marry Jemani Alchin-Boller, I would have been pretty stoked." To Jem, standing by his side, he said, "I'm so proud of you, babe. You are beautiful and smart and you lift people's spirits just by being around them. I hope Gracie grows up to be just like you."

♥　♥　♥

Grace Madeleine Sherson was asleep in her portable cot at the beach apartment while most of the wedding festivities unfolded. She didn't know her mum and aunt danced the night away in peppermint-coloured jandals or that her dad shared proud stories with his friends about how she walked at nine months. She had no idea of the importance of the day she had attended. But she knew people were happy. And she loved her pretty dress. Two weeks later she would wear the same dress for her first birthday party for which her mother and the senior flower girl, Amelia, would make her a ladybird cake with bright red and black icing and chocolate balls for eyes.

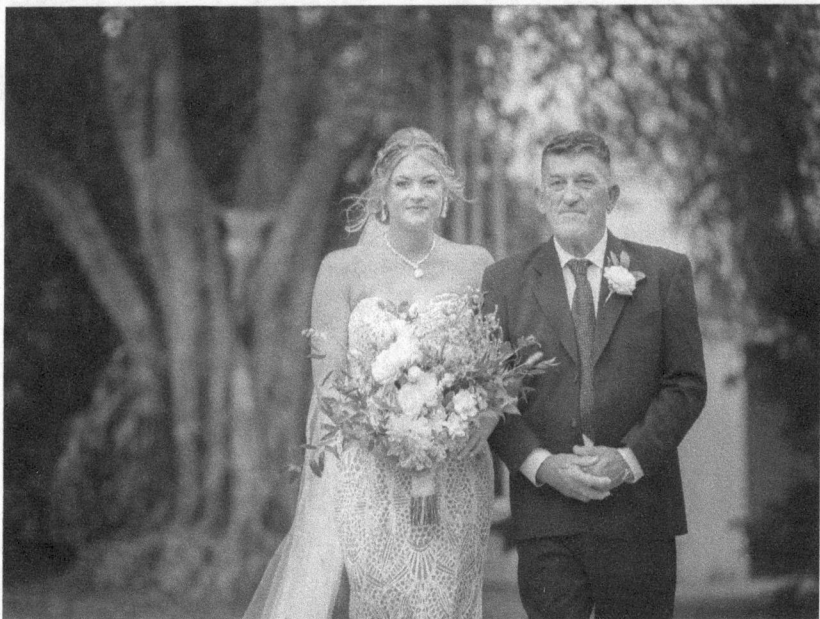

Jem walks down the aisle with her dad, Henry, to the sounds of Amazing Grace.

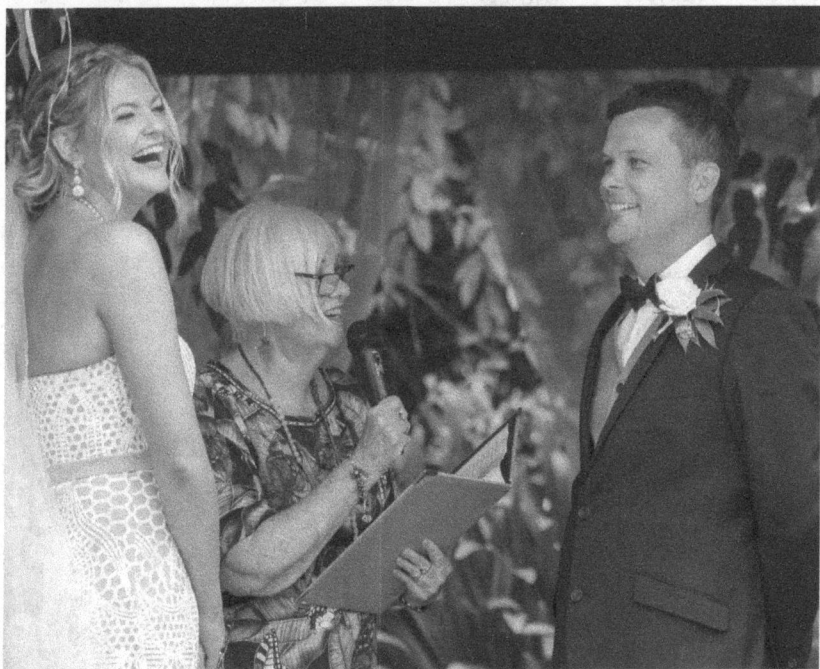

Celebrant Denise Irvine enjoys a light-hearted moment with the couple.
Photo: Agape Photography

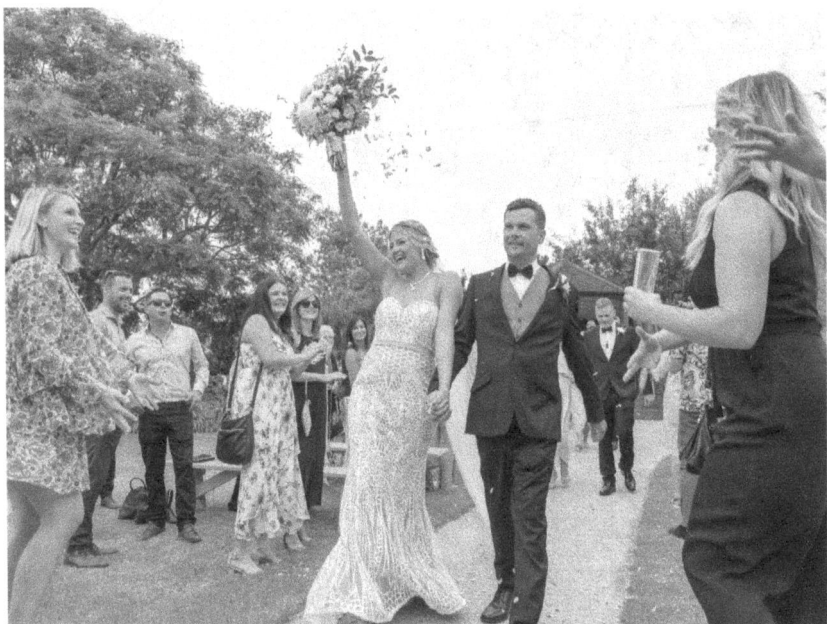

"We did it, babe." Jem and Mark celebrate after their wedding ceremony in Tauranga.

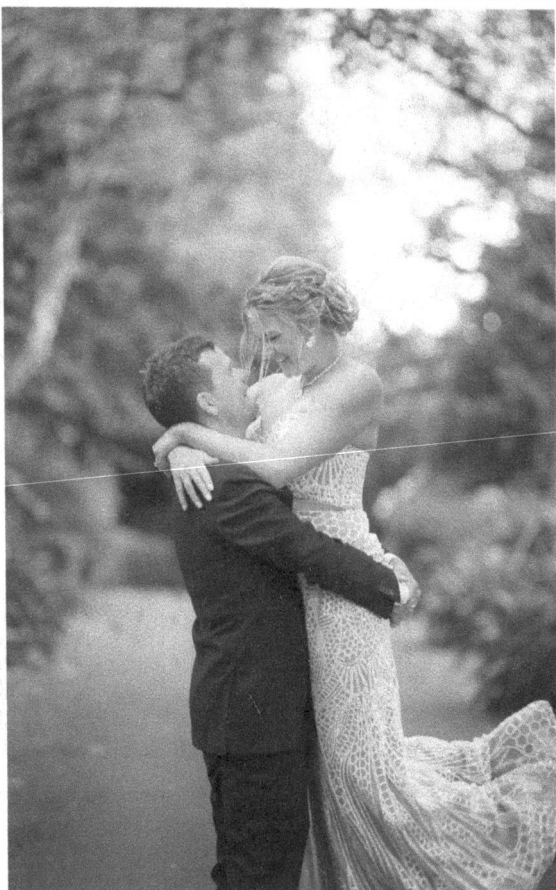

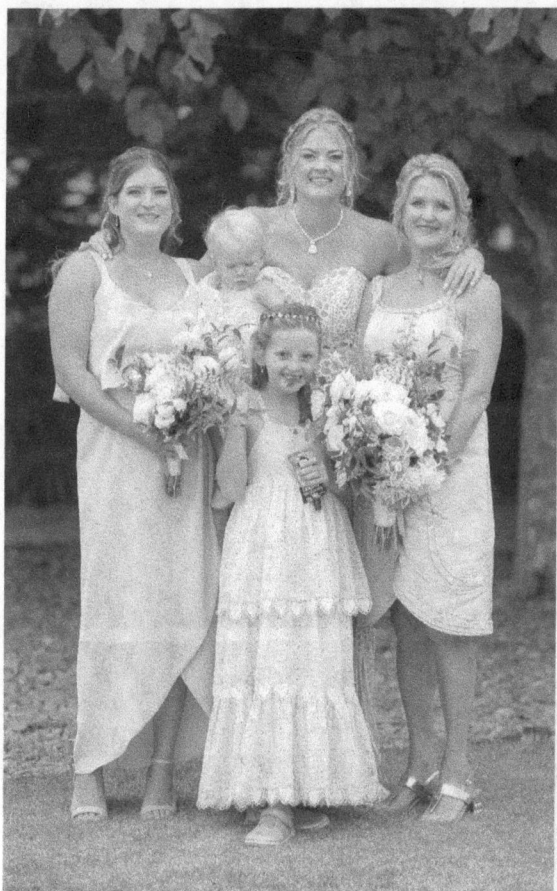

LEFT: The Alchin women, including youngest member, Grace.

BELOW: The families who helped make Grace. From left, Mark with Grace, Jem with Harry, Amelia, Maddy with Lachie and Joe.

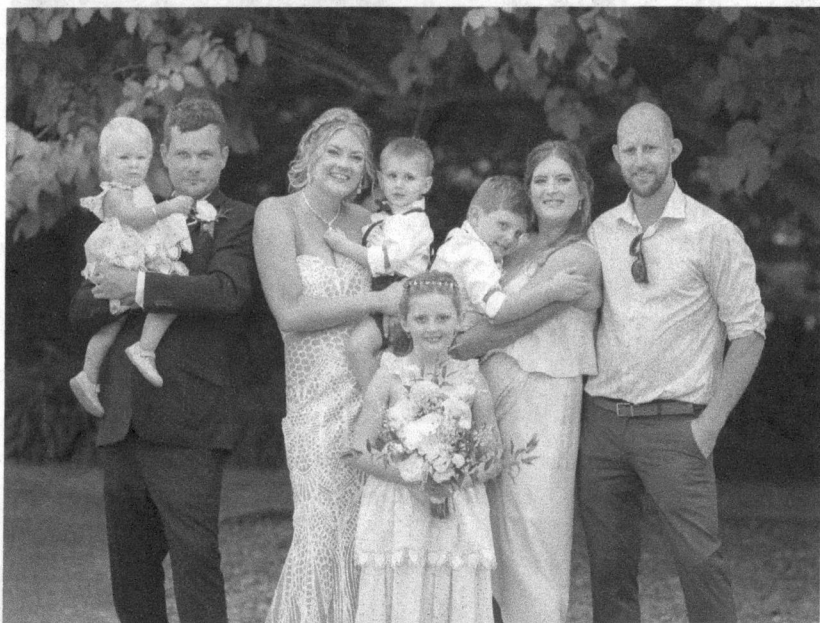

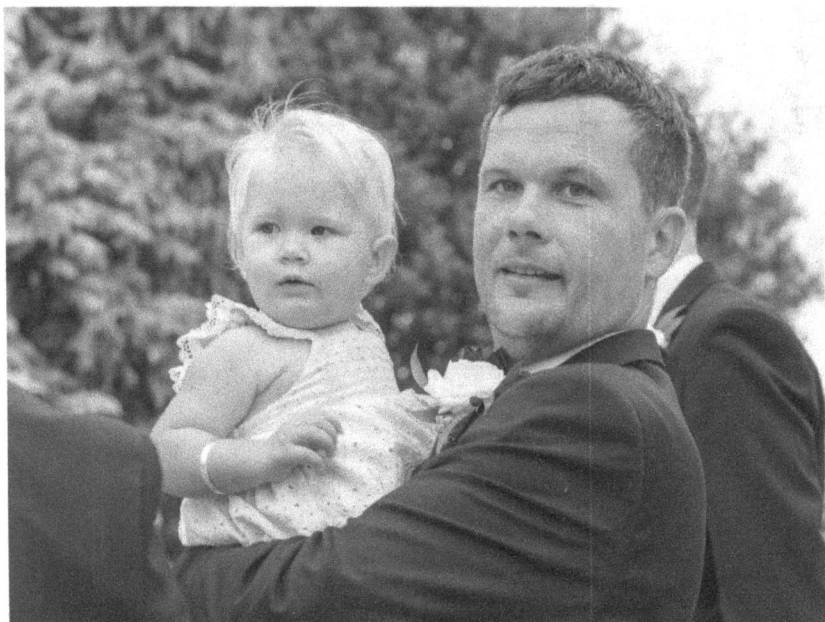

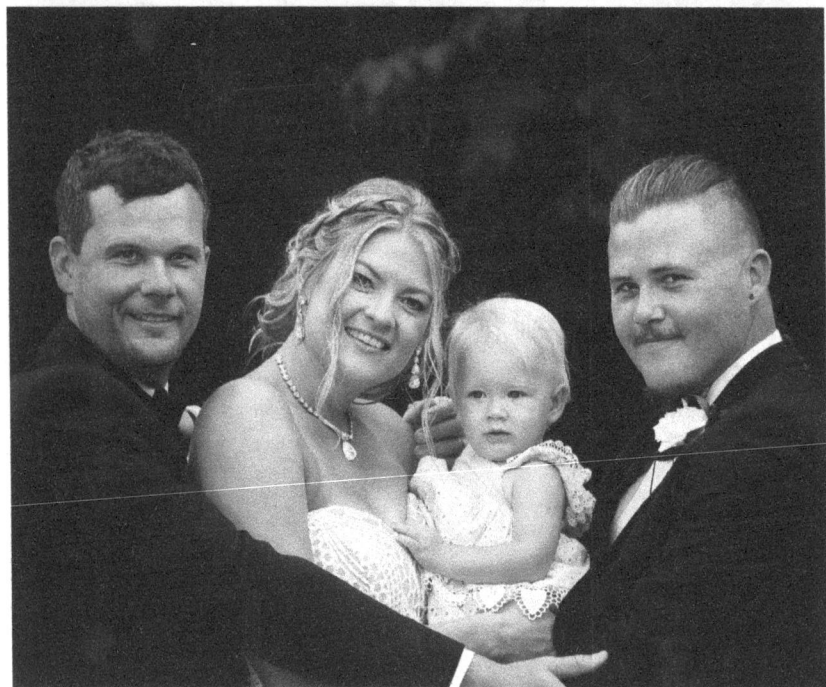

"Family is like the wind: instinctive, raw, fragile, beautiful, at times angry, but always unstoppable." ABOVE: Mark with Grace. BELOW: Mark, Jem, Grace and son, Ethan, 20.

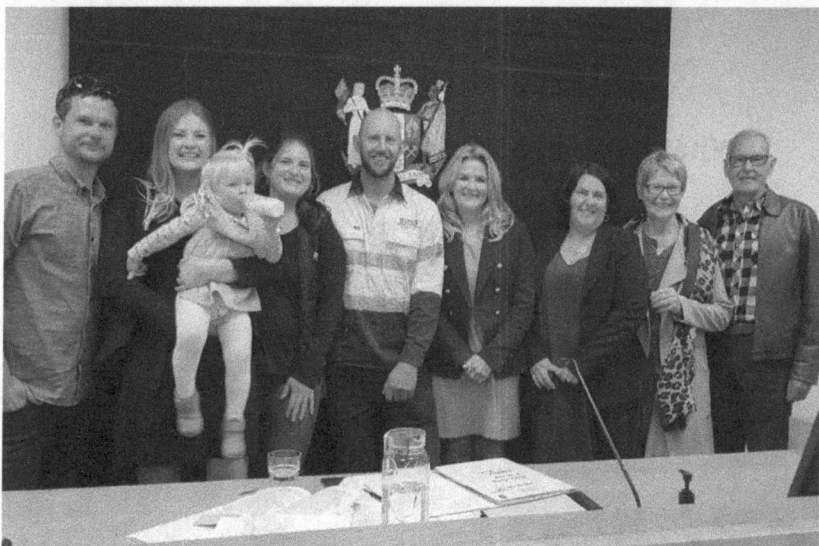

Legally ours. Grace is officially adopted by her biological parents at Hamilton Family Court. From left, Mark, Jem, Grace, Maddy, Joe, Rose, Tracey Gunn, (Jem and Mark's lawyer), Mark's parents, Venetia, and John Sherson. The couples believe the laws relating to adoption in surrogacy need to be changed.

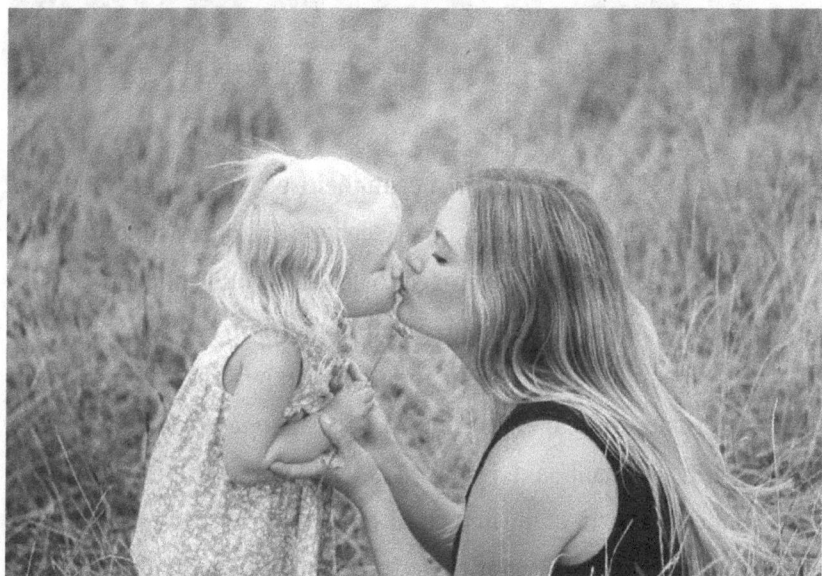

"I love you, mummy." Jem and Grace aged 18 months, share a kiss.

## What happened next?

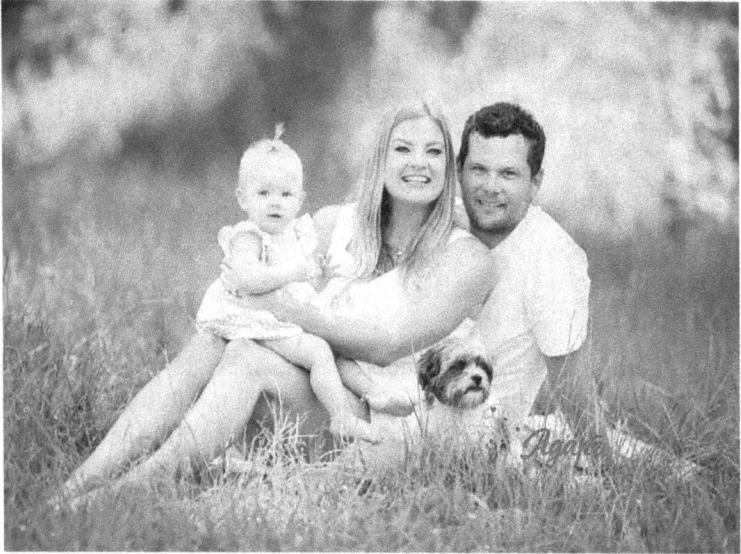

Jem and Mark with Grace, 8 months, and their dog Frankie.

In late 2020, Jem and Mark began their second surrogacy journey. Jem had posted her story on a Facebook surrogacy support group forum, saying how she longed to have a second child. A response came back from Rachael, a young mother of three sons, who had been touched by Jem and Mark's experience. She sent Jem a private message, offering to be a surrogate for their second child. Rachael said, "I have always wanted to be a surrogate since the birth of my first child, but after my other two sons were born I especially want to do it for someone who already has a child, because of how special the sibling relationship is with my own sons."

Jem was blown away. "It was amazing to open this message and have a stranger offering another gift of hope." The two women continued to correspond and their friendship grew. Rachael sent photos of her family on the farm. Her youngest son was then just a year old. Jem loved

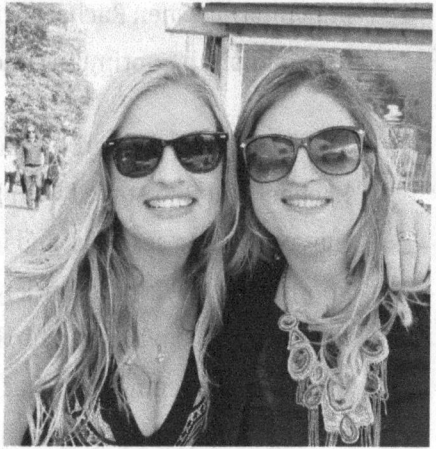

Jem, left, and Maddy. Maddy is overjoyed Jem may have the chance to have a second child.

Rachael's family values, down-to-earth approach, and openness. The couples stayed at each other's homes so they could get to know each other better. Grace helped the boys feed the hens and dig potatoes.

But there were practical issues to consider. Surrogacy is an act of love and generosity, but the logistics have to be managed, especially when the couples live in different parts of the country. Rachael and her husband Ben are sheep and cattle farmers on a property more than three hours from Hamilton. They had to consider how they could undertake counselling with Fertility Associates in Hamilton before ethics committee approval was given. There were other issues, including the lead-up to

161

implantation when Rachael would have to have daily blood tests to establish the optimum time for a successful implantation.

The couples remained undaunted. Everything was possible. Rachael and Ben stayed with Jem and Mark as they underwent the counselling sessions, and in June 2021, their application was approved by E-Cart. In anticipation of another opportunity to have a child, Jem had had further eggs extracted and two viable embryos had been frozen. Rachael started to plan the best time to begin the procedure. If it is successful, Grace could have a brother or sister by the middle of 2022.

Maddy is overjoyed that her sister will have the chance to have a second child. Her decision to carry a baby for Jem and Mark was a result of her close bond with her sister. She is in awe of women who step forward to enable others to have a family.

## Where to get help

There are many helpful websites and social media platforms that connect those interested in surrogacy, including private forums where potential surrogates can make contact with intending parents. These are pages Jem follows on Facebook:

› **NZ IVF, Surrogacy, Donorship, Adoption Support**
   www.facebook.com/groups/238922656741514

› **Breastfeeding Support – La Leche League New Zealand**
   www.facebook.com/LLLNZ

› **Breastfeedingnz – Community organisation**
   https://www.facebook.com/breastfeedingnz

› **Mothers Circle**
   www.facebook.com/motherscirclenz

## Other websites Jem found helpful:

### Breastfeeding

› www.asklenore.info/breastfeeding/induced_lactation/
   protocols4print.shtml

› www.asklenore.info/breastfeeding/induced_lactation/gn_
   protocols.shtml

› kellymom.com/ages/adopt-relactate/relactation-resources/

> www.amazon.com/Breastfeeding-Without-Birthing-Surrogacy-Circumstances/dp/193980700X
(This book "Breastfeeding Without Birthing" was Jem's absolute go-to guide)

> www.canadianbreastfeedingfoundation.org/induced/regular_protocol.shtml

> lalecheleague.org.nz

## Homebirth

> homebirth.org.nz

> nzhistory.govt.nz/women-together/home-birth-associations

## Early parenthood

> www.penguin.co.nz/books/rants-in-the-dark-9780143770183

## New Zealand laws are changing

### Adoption

For some time, there has been widespread agreement that the laws relating to surrogacy in New Zealand are outdated. One of those is the **Adoption Act 1955**. Currently, children born to a surrogate mother are the legal children of that woman even if they share no genetics. The biological parents must apply for an Adoption Order through the Family Court, which can take weeks or months. Without an Adoption Order, a child will have no inheritance rights and the biological parents will have no authority as their parents.

In 2018, after broadcaster Toni Street talked about the difficulties of adopting her biological son born via a surrogate, Prime Minister Jacinda Ardern posted a note on Street's Instagram page, saying changes to the Adoption Act were on the Government's to-do list.

On June 18, 2021, Justice Minister Kris Faafoi announced New Zealand's adoption laws would be reviewed. Public views are being sought on options for change to the **Adoption Act 1955**. To view the discussion document, go to:

› www.justice.govt.nz/assets/Documents/Publications/Adoption-in-Aotearoa-NZ-Discussion-doc.pdf

The work sits alongside a review of surrogacy laws by the Law Commission.

**Surrogacy**

In November 2020, the New Zealand Law Commission, Te Aka Matua o te Ture, began a review of surrogacy law, regulations, and practice in New Zealand. The Commission will look at how the adoption process operates in surrogacy arrangements and consider whether there should be a different process for intending parents to become legal parents. Included in the review are:

» how the law should address any surrogacy matters of particular concern to Māori;

» how surrogacy arrangements should be regulated;

» whether the types of payments intending parents can make under a surrogacy arrangement should be expanded and, if so, what types of payments should be permitted;

» how the law should attribute legal parenthood in surrogacy arrangements;

» how international surrogacy arrangements (where either the intending parent(s) or the surrogate live overseas) should be provided for in Aotearoa New Zealand law; and

» what information should be available to children born from surrogacy arrangements.

The commission will report to the Justice Minister in 2022.

For more information, visit surrogacyreview.nz

## Private Member's Bill

In December 2019, MP Tāmati Coffey, father of a child born through surrogacy, lodged a private member's bill. The Improving Arrangements for Surrogacy Bill includes amendments to five Acts and two sets of Regulations. If it is selected through a ballot or adopted as legislation by the Government, it would address most of the concerns raised, including:

» Enabling surrogates to claim payment for actual and reasonable expenses.

» The establishment of a register to facilitate arrangements between willing women and intending parents.

» If a child is born in an arrangement subject to a court order, the surrogate would cease to be the parent from birth, removing the need for adoption.

For more information on the private member's bill, visit:

www.facebook.com/watch/live/?v=737801576703515

or

www.tvnz.co.nz/one-news/new-zealand/labour-mp-t-mati-coffey-using-his-personal-experience-fight-change-in-surrogacy-laws